Pre- *and* Perinatal
Massage Therapy

A Comprehensive Practitioners' Guide to
♦ Pregnancy   ♦ Labor   ♦ Postpartum

Carole Osborne-Sheets
Integrative Body Therapist

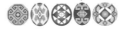

Forward by Judith Aston

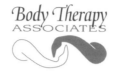
First edition 1998
ISBN #0-9665585-0-2
Second Printing, 1999
Third Printing, 2002
Fourth Printing, 2004

copyright© 1998 by Carole Osborne-Sheets

Birth Symbols designed by Sue Bair.
Illustrations adapted by Sue Bair and Andy Sheets from LifeART Super Anatomy Collections #1 and #3 images. Copyright© 1991-95 TechPool Studies, Inc., USA. Used with permission.

Cover photography and photos on pgs. 10, 18, 31, 37, 66-68, 74, 75, 84, 85, 91, 114, 117, 142 by Jeff Tippet. Harriette Hartigan, pgs. 21, 127. Other photos used with permission of subjects.

The contents of this book have been reviewed and checked for accuracy and appropriateness by a medical doctor, a midwife, childbirth educators, massage therapists, and a physical therapist. However, the author, editor, reviewers, and publisher disclaim all responsibility arising from any errors or adverse effects or results that occur or might occur as a result of the inappropriate application of any of the information contained in this book. Therapeutic massage and bodywork are not a substitute for appropriate medical and prenatal care. It is essential that all pregnant women receive regular professional care, including examinations, monitoring, diagnosis, treatment plans, education, and support for themselves and their babies. If you have a questions or concern about the appropriateness or application of the methods described in this book, consult a prenatal health care professional.

Contents

THE BIRTH SYMBOLS

This book's cover and chapter symbols are computer-generated versions of traditional birth symbols. Women's hands have woven these sometimes simple, often elegant, patterns into textiles and other art in Europe, Asia, Indonesia, and the Philippines for over 400 generations. The diamond shape at their center depicts feminine sexuality enclosing a smaller representation of the child within, with arm and leg-like lines projecting from the sides. It is still the most frequently occurring iconic motif rendered in Eurasian and Indonesian art.

Concept developed from Max Allen
The Birth Symbol in Traditional Women's Art from Eurasia and the Western Pacific
Toronto: The Museum for Textiles, 1981

The book is dedicated to Josh and Elizabeth, whose gestations, births, and lives inspired and continue to influence my work. And to Andy, whose love and willingness to "make it so" sustain me.

♦ ♦ ♦ ♦

INTRODUCTION

It is a privilege to introduce a book that I believe will become an indispensable reference for massage therapists and other health professionals who work with women during the pregnancy, childbirth, and postpartum phases.

In this book, Carole Osborne-Sheets demonstrates her knowledge from many years of study, practice, teaching, and research. The information she imparts to the reader is extensive and covers the relevant aspects of massage in relationship to anatomy, physiology, precautions, and contraindications. She also suggests options for using complementary techniques, including Tai Chi, acupressure, reflexology, and exercise.

In employing these complementary techniques, Osborne-Sheets not only addresses the *physical* body in her recommendations, but frequently reminds the reader to be aware of and sensitive to the emotional needs of the client as well. She encourages the therapist to be well-rounded in therapeutic skills and to always consider the "whole person" in applying these techniques.

The information in the book is organized in a way that *captures* interest; while at the same time manages to effectively educate the reader. It is obvious to the health professional that the main objective of this work is to help the client; this book allows the therapist to better match that *intent* with *ability*.

Judith Aston
Lake Tahoe, Nevada
April, 1998

Acknowledgments

"It takes a village to raise a child," and to create a book.
My sincerest gratitude for their invaluable contributions to this book goes to:

My clients whose pregnancies, births, and/or postpartum experiences have been the context and motivation for my exploring the possibilities of pre- and perinatal massage therapy. Special thanks to those pregnant clients and friends with whom I began this mothering journey, many of whose evocative photographs so aptly give personal texture to this text: Lynn Sharpe-Underwood, Anita Dancoft, Lori Tennant, Rose Pope, Kathleen Estabrook, Kimberly Juntunen, Donna Seda, and Michele Lyons;

My collegues with whom I have brainstormed, experimented, and collaborated on maternity massage at various times since 1979, particularly Sandy Karst, Ed Maupin,Ph.D., Bill Helm, Kate Jordan, Diana Panara, and Ray Hruby, D.O.;

My therapeutic massage and bodywork students whose learning continues to refine my teaching and expressive skills;

The various perinatal healthcare professionals whose technical and medical input has ensured my accuracy and infused a positive perspective into this book, particularly James Webber, M.D.; Diane Smith, midwife; Eliot Cohen, licensed acupuncturist; Jan Neeb, Bradley childbirth instructor; Penny Simkin, P.T, doula trainer; and Liz Smith, prenatal anatomy and physiology instructor;

My teaching assistants and manuscript readers who generated invaluable feedback and bright insights to improve text readability and clarity, especially Linda Hickey, Liz Ellis, Bridget Scadeng, Jan Saunders, and Jennifer Hicks;

Judith Aston for her positive, personal support and introduction;

My family and friends whose patience, perspective, and unconditional love sustained me through the eight long years of gestation, abortion, gestation, many transitions and painful turmoil, and who tolerated more neglect than they deserved in order to bring this book from idea to reality. Special thanks to Andy, Josh, Elizabeth, Mama, Daddy, Linda, Diana, Lori, and Clarissa;

Kathy Sartain, my administrative assistant, whose efficient, positive hard work made this project possible and kept my workshop business running in the meantime;

Jeanne Sapp, my copyeditor, who made good information into better sentences;

Sue Bair, my graphic designer and publishing coordinator, who transformed my words and visions into reality.

FOREWORD

Throughout our history, human hands have woven the fabrics, shaped the vessels, nurtured the food, and cared for the individuals of our families and our communities. Nurturing, knowledgeable tactile communication has been vital to childbearing in most cultures for thousands of years. Aruvedic medical manuals of India detail therapists' instructions for rubbing specially formulated oils into pregnant patients' stretched abdominal skin. Traditional sculptures depict Eskimo fathers supporting and lovingly stroking their wives' backs as attendants assist in the birth. Women who give birth in certain Irish hospitals are held and stroked by a doula (labor assistant) or midwife through most of their notably short, uncomplicated labors. For millions of women, over thousands of years, touch has provided loving support and eased child-bearing discomforts.

During this century, birthing has become increasingly medically managed, especially in many Western societies. While obstetrical innovations have reduced many perinatal risks, the texture of birthing, one of life's most touching, female experiences, has become less tactile and less woman-centered. Recently, however, pregnancy is being reinstated as a natural part of women's reproductive cycle, rather than regarded as a disease or medical condition, unless complications occur. My growth as a pre- and perinatal massage therapist reflects this trend.

In 1979, many in my circle of women friends were pregnant, including me, and I began seeing my first pregnant clients who were elated, yet uncomfortable. Although I'd been practicing bodywork for five years, I was unfamiliar with childbearing so I began some initial research. I quickly confirmed that, with little documented ration-ale, Swedish massage was contraindicated during pregnancy. None of the few, dated textbooks nor the 14, mostly unregulated, U.S. massage therapy schools, including the one I had co-founded, offered any meaningful prenatal curriculum. I'd had little prenatal education, either from my structural balancing apprenticeship, or from my other deep tissue and passive movement studies. More experienced bodyworkers or perinatal specialists, aside from midwives who instinctively touched their laboring women, were unable to provide meaningful guidance. However, my friends', my clients' and my own tired, tight lower back and swollen ankles were delivering a different, most compelling message: pregnant bodies need the structural, physiological, and emotional care of knowledgable touch.

So I was both personally and professionally compelled to expand my research, experimenting on consenting friends, clients, and myself. Collaborating with perinatal professionals and other interested colleagues, I carefully established protocols and guidelines to safely, effectively work with pregnant women. Regular structural work and circulatory massage comforted me and prepared me for labor. The focused, talented touch of my husband and my massage therapist sustained me as I birthed Josh, "the child of my dreams." He transformed me into a mother, and within three months, I co-created and began to teach the first infant massage programs in San Diego to parents and hospital and nursing association staffs.

Over the next few years, between nursing, massaging, and caring for Josh, I expanded my clinical experience with pregnant, laboring, and postpartum women, and I began formulating a prenatal training program for massage therapists and bodyworkers. When I was pregnant four years later and "my precious one," Elizabeth, was born, loving, skillful touch again soothed and attended to me. As my babies grew and our family strengthened, I gradually began teaching maternity massage nationwide. I co-created the original Bodywork for the Childbearing Year® training with Kate Jordan, who was my business partner until 1996. Then I independently refined and expanded that former course into my current workshop, Pre- and Perinatal Massage Therapy. Over these years, I have had the honor of preparing thousands of practitioners throughout the United States and Canada to be perinatal massage specialists.

In contrast to the '70s, many therapeutic massage and bodywork curricula now include introductions to pregnancy massage. Several national programs offer prenatal massage therapy as continuing education. Hospital-based prenatal massage programs are underway. Midwives and physicians refer women for massage therapy. Large, multi-therapist practices specializing in maternity massage are flourishing in several U.S. cities and in Canada. Maternity massage books and commercial videos target both professionals and the pregnant public.

While there is an unprecedented interest in pre- and perinatal massage therapy, I am concerned that the pendulum may have swung from an absolute, somewhat irrational taboo to an equally ill-advised enthusiasm for universal advocacy of maternity massage. With good intentions, therapists with little education or understanding of the intricacies of pregnancy physiology blithely assume pregnancy massage simply necessitates accommodating a large belly. Videos and childbirth educators encourage prenatal and labor massage while offering no substantial safety precautions to well-meaning partners.

I have written this book to provide somatic practitioners the comprehensive theoretical foundation necessary to safely weave appropriate therapeutic touch back into maternity healthcare. It is primarily addressed to these "touch specialists" of the healthcare professions: massage therapists, bodyworkers, neuromuscular therapists, Rolfers®, other hands-on practitioners, and physical therapists. It is also the intention of this book to provide midwives, nurse-midwives, obstetrical nurses, physicians, and childbirth educators the background to responsibly include skilled touch as an adjunct to their patient care.

Personal examples from pregnant women and from practitioners' clinical experiences elaborate an overview of research documenting the meaningful benefits of therapeutic massage and bodywork throughout pregnancy and labor, and in the postpartum period. Physiological, structural, and emotional developments in the childbearing year are explained, emphasizing ramifications for somatic practices. General guidelines for effective, safe therapy are presented, with specific contraindications and precautions relevant to each trimester and to most forms of Western touch therapies. Precautions are detailed for appropriate work when complications and high-risk pregnancies occur. This theoretical foundation will prepare practitioners to knowledgeably modify their work.

Detailed instructions provide a limited but effective number of essential techniques for each trimester of pregnancy, for labor preparation and facilitation, and for postpartum recovery. I feel that hands-on techniques are best learned by demonstration and supervised practice; therefore, only selected techniques, essential to addressing women's childbearing needs, are detailed, although meaningful guidelines for addressing specific physiologic, postural, and psychological concerns are explained. This book will best be utilized in conjunction with hands-on training, such as my Pre-and Perinatal Massage Therapy certification workshop.

Britain's noted childbirth educator and author, Sheila Kitzinger introduces her powerful anthropological survey, *Ourselves as Mothers*, with this statement:

"To be a mother is to take on one of the most emotionally and intellectually demanding, exasperating, strenuous, anxiety-arousing, and deeply satisfying tasks that any human being can undertake."

To all practitioners reading this book, I'd like to add:

To nurture the birth of a mother and of her baby with skilled touch is one of the most intellectually challenging, emotionally and physically demanding, humbling, inspiring, and life-enhancing experiences that a somatic practitioner can engage in. Appropriate touch with childbearing women has the potential to positively change not only individual women and their families, but also to knit an ever-widening fabric of nurturing touch to help unite and transform our current violent, touch-aversive societies.

Carole Osborne-Sheets
San Diego, CA
June, 1998

Chapter

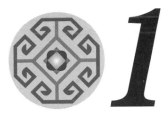

1

Benefits of Pre- and Perinatal Massage Therapy

"In my high-risk situation, I don't know if I hadn't received the massage work if I would have carried to full term. That is, of course, impossible to determine, but I definitely feel that the pregnancy went along much more smoothly and comfortably, and the recovery was much quicker than with my previous pregnancies." — Jennifer

*P*regnancy creates significant physiological, structural, psychological, relational, and spiritual changes in a woman's life. For many, the perinatal period, from gestational week 32 until two weeks after childbearing, is tumultuous. Massage therapy, bodywork, and other somatic practices are particularly effective forms of adjunctive healthcare during this time, offering a wide range of benefits to the expectant mother and her baby.

STRESS REDUCTION AND RELAXATION

Pregnancy — a time of transitions

While pregnancy is a welcome blessing for most, it can bring with it many changes. As her body transforms, a woman must adjust to her altered physiologic functioning. Her pregnant body is not only shaped differently, but her gait and other movement patterns may alter to accommodate her enlarging uterus and breasts. As her hair changes texture and her skin darkens in several areas, she may feel as though she is no longer her former physical self.

Pregnancy is often a time of emotional upheaval and anxiety, as well as a time of euphoria and joy. In a single day a pregnant woman's emotions may fluctuate from profound love, triumph, glee, and fulfillment to anger, fear, doubt, isolation, and worry. Her relationships with her mate, parents, friends, and co-workers change. Life issues that may have been repressed sometimes surface during pregnancy, including the legacies of physical and emotional abuse. Renegotiations of her degree of dependence, interdependence, and her sense of her societal roles often arise at this time. A new baby destabilizes a woman's financial outlook and strains low- and middle-income families' abilities to make ends meet. At a time when every woman needs support, many American women find themselves isolated, without the community and familial support of former times and of other cultures. An alarming number of women also suffer abuse from their spouses.[1]

With more birth control and lifestyle options available in recent years, women have more apparent control and greater expectations of pregnancy. Since the 1980s, more women delay pregnancy until their later twenties, thirties, or even into their forties.[2,3] Many women choose to have only one or two children and are more deliberate in the timing of their pregnancies. This can result in pregnancies with greater significance and investment of emotional energy.

Popular media images create parental expectations of childbearing as a romantic, blissful time. Childbirth education and other instructional program materials may cause an increase in performance anxiety. Consequently, some parents expect an "ideal" birth and anguish over anything that falls short of their expectations. Others cling to real or imagined promises of painless, risk-free labor, and trust technology and pharmaceuticals to assuage their fears about the upcoming birth. Health issues, such as diabetes or poor nutrition, increase maternal and fetal risks in some pregnancies so that these women are more apprehensive about the pregnancy's outcome.

With all of these concerns, pregnant women will usually experience increased stress. Stress activates the sympathetic branch of the autonomic nervous system.

While useful in responding to an emergency, such as applying the car brakes to avoid an accident, or catching a falling child, chronic sympathetic arousal provoked by worries and anxieties can have significant negative impacts on childbearing and development.

Ongoing stress increases adrenal production of stress hormones, creating a freeze, fight, or flight response.[4] Research reveals that stress has many deleterious effects pre- and perinatally including:

♦ increased maternal heart rate, blood pressure, vomiting, nausea, spontaneous abortion, toxemia, and immune system dysfunction

♦ reduced blood supply to uterus, by as much as 65%, resulting in lower fetal heart rate and reduced blood oxygenation

♦ interference with fetal brain and central nervous system development

♦ higher incidence of miscarriage, prematurity, prolonged labors with more complications, and postpartum complications

♦ increased perinatal fetal distress, low birth weight, and infant irritability, restlessness, crying, and digestive disturbances [5, 6]

Recent animal studies suggest that effects of prenatal stress may reverberate far into a child's life. At the University of Wisconsin's Harlow Primate Laboratory, adolescent Rhesus monkeys whose mothers were stressed during their pregnancies were not only more anxious, clumsier, sicker, and shier than control teen monkeys; they were also slower to learn and unable to focus on tasks. Researchers speculated that their results might offer clues to one of the causes of attention deficit disorder (ADD) in children.[7]

"Massage therapy is very relaxing. I hadn't done much for myself since I became pregnant, and I can really see how it benefits me and my baby by loosening muscles and making me slow down." — Melissa

Support, relaxation, and prenatal massage therapy

*I*ndividualized hands-on time with a somatic practitioner presents a unique and potent experience of support and relaxation for pregnant women. Support is defined as "anything that makes a person feel good, function more effectively, or be more optimistic."[8] "Relaxation is characterized by turning inward, by concentrating on one's own body and mind rather than on external events. Inherent in the relaxed state is a certain feeling of detachment; that is, a lack of concern for how one is doing...thus people do not so much 'do' relaxation as permit it to happen. They merely let go and allow relaxation to take place."[9]

In contrast to the effects of stress, support and relaxation activate the parasympathetic branch of the autonomic nervous system, increasing steroid

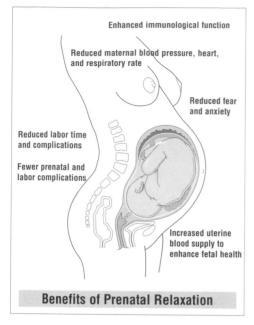

Enhanced immunological function

Reduced maternal blood pressure, heart, and respiratory rate

Reduced fear and anxiety

Reduced labor time and complications

Fewer prenatal and labor complications

Increased uterine blood supply to enhance fetal health

Benefits of Prenatal Relaxation

production. This helps create balance in the body and encourages a healthy, smoothly functioning state, characterized by steady blood pressure, pulse, and respiratory rate; regular blood flow to uterus, placenta, and fetus; healthy immune system functioning, emotional states, and response to stressful stimuli; and reduced fear and anxiety.[10]

An overview of research indicates that support can counteract the negative effects of stress. Most notable of these studies was the work done in 1972 by Katherine Nuckolls of Yale Nursing School. She studied several hundred pregnant women who had a number of life changes in the two years immediately preceding and/or during their pregnancy, such as death of a family member; crisis in relationships, finances, or health; or changes in jobs or homes. She found that those who also had strong support systems had one-third the complications of those who experienced similar stresses without a support system.[11]

Learning how to relax is an integral part of all childbirth education programs. Regardless of methods, all childbirth experts agree on the positive results of relaxation — increased well-being for both mother and baby and increased chances for a positive birth experience. Progressive relaxation, visualization, autogenic training, meditation, and other relaxation techniques reduce stress during pregnancy, help relieve pain and anxiety during labor and birth, and assist in coping with the challenging days and years of parenting.[12, 13, 14]

Massage therapy also can be profoundly relaxing. In fact, there is documented evidence that massage therapy applications as brief as six to twenty minutes in length produce muscle relaxation.[15, 16, 17] Recent studies at the Touch Research Institute involving sexually abused women showed promising results as well. Immediately after receiving 30-minute massages, twice weekly for one month, subjects reported feeling less depressed and anxious. Their decreased salivary cortisol levels (primary stress hormones) confirmed their perceptions. Over the study period, these women experienced a decrease in depression and in life-event stress. While sexually abused women in a control group practicing relaxation therapy also reported less anxiety and depression, their stress hormones did not change, and they reported an increasingly negative attitude toward touch.[18]

Massage can provide an experience of "letting go" and focusing inwardly, and it can create the same positive physiologic states and increased alpha brain wave activity as meditation. Variations in pressure, rhythm, and positioning flood the sensory nerve pathways with input that can increase body awareness and override signals of pain and stress.[19]

Research at the University of North Texas in 1988 specifically documented the effectiveness of massage therapy with chronic pain patients. Patients who were experiencing chronic headache and back pain were massaged twice weekly for four weeks. When compared to control patients, they experienced significant reduction of physiological pain, fatigue, and depression; improvement in mood and vitality; reduction in muscle tension and perception of tension; and decreased levels of mental and physical strain.[20]

A massage practitioner provides soothing, nurturing touch combined with focused, individualized attention to the pregnant woman's physical and emotional concerns. This regular, caring contact can be a vital component of a pregnant woman's support system, especially when family and friends are not providing such support. Practitioners with complementary skills and training in counseling and emotional processing can offer attentive, nonjudgmental listening. This presents additional opportunities for helping women to understand and assimilate the strong emotional states common during pregnancy. Practitioners can also educate women in body-use that assists in managing and reducing stress. They provide well-researched referrals to other professionals dealing with pre- and perinatal health and emotional well-being.

Prenatal Massage Therapy = Stress Reduction

Somatic Practitioners provide:

Nurturing, skilled touch

Individualized attention to needs

Emotional support, especially in the absence of supportive family and friends

Attentive, nonjudgmental listening and emotional processing

Education and encouragement in stress-reducing activities

Appropriate referrals to other perinatal specialists

For labor preparation, prenatal specialists Nancy and Mike Samuels recommend women practice deep sustained levels of relaxation for 45-60 minutes without falling asleep, especially in the last six to eight weeks of pregnancy.[21] This is the exact length of most massage therapy sessions. Additionally, massage therapy is received in an environment that is most conducive to relaxation; in a comfortable position allowing the muscles to relax; with a passive attitude that allows relaxation to take place; in a quiet place in which one won't be disturbed and where a deep, regular rate of breathing can be encouraged and sustained.

CIRCULATORY BENEFITS

*T*o provide for fetal needs, prenatal adaptations of the circulatory system are profound. Resulting discomforts, such as edema, varicose veins, and high blood pressure, often respond well to appropriate massage therapy.

Elevated estrogen and progesterone production during pregnancy increases total blood volume by as much as 30% to 50%. By weeks 24 to 34, the plasma volume alone has increased by 40%. All blood components, including white blood cells, serum protein, and serum enzymes, are elevated. Since red blood cells increase at a lower rate, many women become anemic. Perhaps the greatest change women notice is the increase in interstitial fluid volume (edema), which is 40% higher than non-pregnant levels in the third trimester and results in swollen legs and ankles.

Pelvic myofascial restriction and the mechanical effects of the weighty uterus contribute to swelling, working much like a cork in a bottle of effervescent liquid, restricting femoral fluid return. As a result, about 75% of women suffer normal, pregnancy-induced (non-pitting) edema in the lower extremities, first occurring in the late second or third trimester.

Uterine compression of the iliac veins and inferior vena cava also restricts blood flow contributing to the development of varicose veins in the legs and vulva. Increased femoral venous blood pressure challenges the integrity of the valves of the femoral, saphenous, and other leg veins already compromised by progesterone's relaxation of the smooth muscle walls. A woman's heredity and diet, prolonged sitting or standing, and the position and size of her baby are important factors contributing to edema and varicose veins. Higher levels of progesterone also dilate the peripheral blood vessels that often burst to form spider veins (spider nevi).

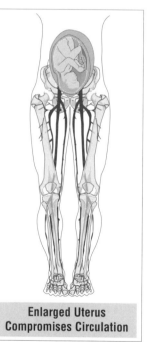

Enlarged Uterus Compromises Circulation

Swelling in the hands, face, or the entire body, or that which occurs in the first or second trimester may be indicative of a complication of pregnancy called gestational edema proteinurea hypertension complex (GEPH). (See hypertensive disorders, Chapter 2.) This complication is also known as preeclampsia and is typified by pitting edema, as evidenced by a depression and blanching of the skin for several seconds to several minutes after it is pressed.

As indicated by the name, GEPH also is typified by high blood pressure. While arterial blood pressure usually remains constant prenatally, when pregnancy-induced hypertension (PIH) occurs it involves an increase of 30 systolic or 15 diastolic readings (systolic/diastolic). For a small percentage of women, edema can result in carpal tunnel syndrome with moderate to severe pain in the arms and hands, particularly in the middle and index fingers.

> *"Before the massage, I had been holding water in my legs and feet. Afterwards, the swelling lessened, and my whole body felt very relaxed and ready for a peaceful nap."* — Aletha

Swedish massage and lymphatic drainage massage produce autonomic vascular reflexes that promote delivery of oxygen and nutrients and removal of waste materials.[22] Manually pumped by effleurage, petrissage, kneading, and other compression techniques, lymph capillaries are repeatedly emptied and refilled, producing a sustained increase in the rate of lymph formation and removal. Massage also opens capillary beds, which increases the total capillary surface area and temporarily increases both venous and capillary hydrostatic pressure to increase lymph filtration and formation.[23]

Specifically for the pregnant woman, this effect facilitates the physiological processes of gestation. An enhanced supply of nutrients and oxygen and accelerated removal of waste products promotes cellular respiration, improving both mother's and baby's tissue health. Techniques promoting circulation of blood and lymph, especially Swedish massage and lymphatic drainage techniques, support circulatory function. These methods decrease the negative effects of increased blood and interstitial fluid volumes.

These same circulatory techniques assist in reducing edema. Performed rhythmically, lymphatic strokes work like a hydraulic pump shifting excess fluid from the tissues to the blood.[24] The mechanical effects of compression strokes increase capillary blood flow and produce local vasodilatation through increased histamine release. These effects also may be induced through the autonomic vascular reflexes described above.[25]

If myofascial restriction in the inguinal area is contributing to leg edema and varicose veins, careful, specific deep tissue and/or passive movement techniques can help relieve edema. Most benefit is derived from gentle work with the hip joints, tensor fasciae latae, rectus femoris, sartorius, and adductor muscles, and the inguinal ligament. (See circulatory system precautions, Chapter 2.)

Studies indicate that slow, rhythmic stroking paravertebrally from the crown of the head to the sacral area lowers high blood pressure and heart rate.[26, 27] Any other methods that promote parasympathetic activity should lower blood pressure as well.

Effects of Swedish Massage and Lymphatic Drainage During Pregnancy:

Assist in reducing edema

Reduce varicose vein development and pain

Promote increased blood and lymph circulation

Open capillary beds

Promote cellular respiration

Reduce blood pressure

IMPROVED PHYSIOLOGICAL FUNCTIONING

Skin stimulation research

*T*he skin's importance to the human being is evidenced by a few pertinent facts: it is one of the largest organs in the body, measuring 6% to 8% of total body weight, and a quarter-sized area of the skin contains over three million cells, including extensive sensory nerves endings and blood supply.[28] Ashley Montagu, anthropologist and "skin scholar," describes the brain as "the inside layer of the skin, and the skin the outside layer of the brain." This analogy is supported by embryological development, as the skin tissue is the first to differentiate, and it evolves out of the same tissue as the brain.[29]

Research on the far-reaching effects of skin stimulation powerfully argues the potential benefits of pre- and perinatal massage therapy. Many animal studies of this century document the widespread importance of the skin and its stimulation through touch, including licking and stroking. Post-thyroidectomy rats who were stroked and handled by caretakers suffered 13% mortality, as compared to 79% mortality among those receiving routine feeding and cleaning only.[30] Gentled or stroked rats and mice in many other experiments demonstrated differences from non-gentled control groups. Pups of gentled rats and mice opened their eyes sooner after birth, were more active, developed motor coordination earlier, and weighed more at weaning. Stroked animals had stronger immune systems and showed 50% more synaptic junctions. They were more sexually active. Socially more dominant, they were curious, calmer, better problem solvers, and possessed advanced mothering skills.

Their superior motor, mental, and social development lasts their entire lives. These positive results of tactile stimulation increase if the animals are stroked throughout their maturation. The non-gentled control animals in these studies were more excitable, timid, and fearful. They tended toward rage reactions in response to frustration, and they often bit each other and their caretakers.[31-38]

The importance of skin stimulation during pregnancy was demonstrated in studies of pregnant rats. An experimental group wore large collars that restricted their characteristic licking of their swelling abdomens and teats. Reflecting decreased estrogen and prolaclin production, the collared rats' mammary development was 50% less than that of the control rats. These mothers randomly and ineffectively attempted to build their nests, where they delivered fewer live off-spring than control mothers. Their placentas were very poorly developed, reducing placental lactogen and progesterone levels. Avoiding contact with their litters, they neglected cleaning the afterbirth and licking their young. Fewer pups survived the neglect, and their mothers had difficulties in nursing them.[39]

It would appear from these animal studies that:

♦ skin stimulation stimulates the brain and creates positive effects in all body systems; and,

♦ touch during pregnancy promotes secretion of hormones that improve pregnancy outcomes and produce appropriate mothering behaviors.

Massage and other touch therapies inherently provide pregnant, laboring, and postpartum women with these general physiological benefits.

"I had felt like a stitch in my side for weeks. After last session's deeper breathing and those strokes on my ribs, that's gone. Relaxing and breathing to my baby seems to make this all more real to me, too." — Kim

Respiratory benefits of prenatal massage

Specific, well-designed massage therapy can also improve pre- and perinatal respiratory function. Although elevated progesterone production prompts increased exchange of gases with each breath (tidal volume), most expectant women tend to feel short of breath and to hyperventilate. This rapid, shallow, upper chest breathing pattern is the result of the growing uterus restricting diaphragm excursion and a tendency towards anterior rotation of the pectoral girdle. Compensating for the enlarged abdomen and breasts, many women lean back as though to prevent falling forward. This posteriorly shifts the upper thoracic area while the lower ribcage presses more anteriorly, further negatively impacting respiration.

With individual guidance in diaphragmatic or abdominal breathing, the pregnant client can correct shallow, rapid, or paradoxical (abdomen contracts with inhalation, expands with exhalation) breathing patterns. Diaphragmatic breathing promotes relaxation, reduces stress, and relieves musculoskeletal strain on the neck, chest, and upper back caused by inefficient breathing. Although the inferior ribcage circumference expands during pregnancy, instruction in more lateral and posterior ribcage expansion fosters more costal, deeper diaphragmatic breathing patterns.[40]

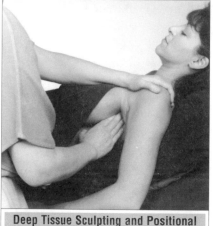

Deep Tissue Sculpting and Positional Relaxation of Pectoralis Minor

Deep tissue massage, structural realignment guidance, passive and active movement, and trigger point therapy all improve breathing by correcting restrictive postural deviations and improving neck, abdomen, and chest mobility.[41] Myofascial restriction, tender points, and habitual holding patterns in the scalenes, sternocleidomastoid, intercostals, pectoralis major and minor, levator scapula, rhomboids, trapezius, and serratus anterior, require particular attention.

Gastrointestinal system benefits

Secondary effects of elevated hormonal levels are partially responsible for many pregnant clients' gastrointestinal complaints. Human chorionic gonadatrophin (hCG) maintains a woman's estrogen levels in early pregnancy, inhibits maternal rejection of the embryo as foreign tissue, and increases basal temperature. It is also suspected to be at least partially responsible for several of the most common pregnancy discomforts: indigestion, heartburn, nausea, and vomiting. While more common in weeks 2 to 14, "morning sickness" continues for some women throughout their pregnancies.

Massage therapy may help counteract the negative nutritional impacts of these conditions. Several studies of premature infants and cocaine-exposed premature infants documented significant weight gain for massaged infants compared to unmassaged control infants. Researchers have proposed the explanation that massage increases vagal nerve activity which stimulates production of food absorption hormones.[42] Extrapolating from these infant studies, a pregnant woman's nutrient utilization may be improved with similar Swedish massage strokes.

Constipation is experienced by 25% of all expectant mothers. Progesterone relaxes the smooth muscles of the digestive system creating lethargic peristaltic activity. Compressed intestines, dislocated posteriorly and laterally by the growing uterus, process food more slowly. The enlarged uterus also presses on both the stomach and the gallbladder, and more than 75% of all women have heartburn, especially in later pregnancy and when lying down.

Unfortunately, the many massage techniques so effective in relieving constipation are not safe during pregnancy. Deep abdominal effleurage, kneading, and vibration create more intrauterine pressure than seems safe during pregnancy; however, reflexive techniques, including foot reflexology (zone therapy) and Eastern-based manual therapies, may positively influence gastrointestinal functioning.[43, 44]

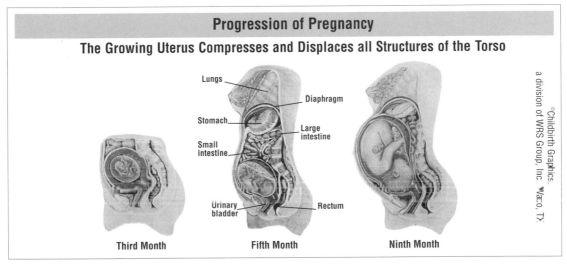

Progression of Pregnancy
The Growing Uterus Compresses and Displaces all Structures of the Torso

Lungs — Diaphragm — Stomach — Large intestine — Small intestine — Urinary bladder — Rectum

Third Month — **Fifth Month** — **Ninth Month**

©Childbirth Graphics, a division of WRS Group, Inc. Waco, TX

Urinary system benefits

Urinary frequency, decreased bladder tone, and longer emptying time are just a few of a pregnant woman's urinary discomforts and dysfunctions. The swelling uterus compresses both the bladder and its ureters, slowing urination and reducing bladder space. Weight gain also strains the pelvic floor muscles, reducing their sphincter and supportive capacities. Urinary output is greater, initially because of hormonal fluctuations, and later in pregnancy as more blood is pumped through the kidneys for filtration. These factors also increase the likelihood of bladder and kidney infections during pregnancy. Many women leak small amounts of urine when laughing, sneezing, or coughing (urinary stress incontinence). This condition may worsen from the inherent stretching and possible damage to the pelvic floor in a vaginal birth.

Though outside the scope of practice of most massage practitioners, partner or self-massage of a woman's pelvic floor muscles readies the area for birthing, as does encouragement of daily, numerous repetitions of Kegel exercises. Tightening pelvic muscles as though stopping urine flow, and doing other strengthening exercises improves their tone and vascularization. Pelvic floor exercise also expands a woman's awareness and control of her pelvic floor, skills which are especially helpful during labor and birth.[45] Reflexive techniques on the feet, hands, and energy meridians may also enhance bladder and kidney function.

REDUCTION OF MUSCULOSKELETAL STRAIN AND PAIN

Prenatal structural balance

*I*n a recent survey, prenatal massage therapists cited relief from musculoskeletal aches and pains as the primary motivator for their clients seeking therapy.[46] More anterior weight in the breasts and abdomen generally challenges a pregnant woman's structural integrity. As pregnancy progresses, her pelvis will tend to anteriorly rotate, spilling the uterus forward against the abdominal walls. This increases the lumbar curvature and stretches the abdominal muscles, usually separating the rectus abdominis at the linea alba (diastus recti) by the third trimester. To compensate, she leans her upper ribcage more posterior, and her head and neck jut forward anterior of the optimal vertical line. These compensations strain all of the posterior musculature creating fatigue, tightness, excessive fibrous buildup (fibrosis), and hyperirritable, tender points that refer pain to distant sites (myofascial trigger points). Her pectoral girdle sags into forward rotation. Increased uterine weight encourages strain to the pelvic floor; external rotation of the hip joint; modifications of iliopsoas function in walking; and causes the characteristic waddling gait of pregnant women. To prevent falling forward with the increased anterior weight, her knees hyperextend, and her calves frequently cramp. She tends to collapse her increased weight into the medial arches of her weary feet.

These postural adjustments and the recommended weight gain of 25-30 pounds both strain and compress the weight-bearing joints and associated myofascial structures identified in the following diagram. Most importantly, the relationship of the ilea and sacrum at the sacroiliac joints shifts when the enlarged abdomen protrudes anteriorly. As the pelvis anteriorly rotates, the ligaments of these deep pelvic joints are compressed, strained, and can become hyper- or hypomobile in response. Lumbosacral joint compression and lumbar and pelvic muscular strain can be severe. The hip joints become compressed and externally rotated. All of these strains are usually multiplied when a woman exceeds the recommended weight gain.

As early as the tenth week of pregnancy, the hormone relaxin begins softening the connective tissue throughout the body in preparation for labor. The resulting laxity in ligaments, tendons, and fascia contributes to joint instability and strain on weightbearing structures, especially in the lumbar spine and pelvis. Many women report feeling as though they have become "a loose goose," ambulating similarly to Dorothy's scarecrow friend in "The Wizard of Oz."

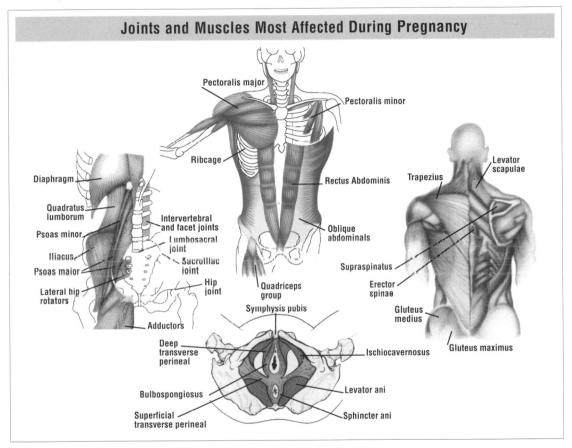

Joints and Muscles Most Affected During Pregnancy

Back and pelvic pain in pregnancy

*M*any women report their first incidence of chronic back pain during pregnancy. Forty-eight percent to 56% of all expectant women experience some back pain, especially during the fifth through the ninth months. Of these women, 50% suffer pain in the sacroiliac area, 25% in the upper back, and 25% in the lower back. Though buttock and posterior thigh pain may occur, only about 1% have true sciatica.[47]

Posturally-induced strain to localized segments of the posterior musculature and ligaments, and referred pain from both posterior and anterior trigger points create concentrated areas of back pain. Poor abdominal tone and diastus recti contribute to back pain. Strained uterine ligaments may refer pain to the pelvis, and relaxin-softened pelvic and spinal ligaments are often achy. A fetus with a preferred uterine position often overburdens the favored side of the mother's back, making it tired and sore from the unbalanced weight load; some women develop temporary scoliosis from fetal positioning preferences.[48]

Clients often describe the generalized back pain of pregnancy as fatigue, tightness, and achiness. Sacroiliac pain is typified by a chronic soreness in the upper, medial quadrant of the buttocks, across the iliac crest, or at the posterior iliac spine of the pelvis and radiating for several inches. Prolonged periods of standing or sitting, wearing high heels, and insufficient back support while seated, can all create strain to these joints softened by relaxin and stressed by any pelvic rotation. Occasionally one sacroiliac joint's hypomobility will result in excessive mobility in the other. A sharp, stabbing posterior pelvic pain may be experienced when the client rolls from a supine position.[49]

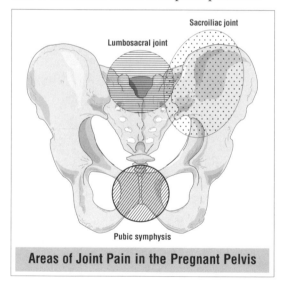

Areas of Joint Pain in the Pregnant Pelvis

Sacroiliac joint

Lumbosacral joint

Pubic symphysis

Pain from other pelvic joints varies with the source. Achiness in the center of the sacral and lumbar areas may indicate strain and compression of the lumbosacral joint. Sharp, stabbing anterior pain in the center of the pelvis, particularly when rolling over or climbing stairs indicates separation of the pubic symphysis. Softened by relaxin, this joint is vulnerable to horizontal sheering strains that are excruciating when movements elevate or depress one side of the pelvis.

The pregnant uterus blossoms from a plum-sized pelvic organ to watermelon proportions. Reaching xiphoid process level by the ninth month, the uterus is suspended by the supportive structure of its eight ligaments. Formed of thickened external uterine connective tissue, these ligaments include:

♦ two broad ligaments proceeding laterally, attached to the internal pelvic cavity walls

♦ two round ligaments extending from the anterior, superior surface of the

uterus, through the inguinal area, and
attached into the connective tissue
of the pubic mons

♦ two sacrouterine ligaments continuing
from the posterior uterus attached to
the posterior pelvic cavity wall and
anterior surface of the sacrum at S2&3

♦ one small anterior ligament attached
to the bladder, and one stretching from
the posterior uterus to the rectum

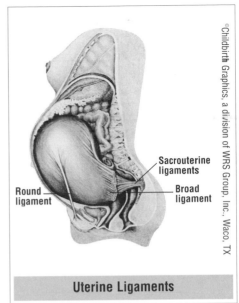

Uterine Ligaments

©Childbirth Graphics, a division of WRS Group, Inc., Waco, TX

As uterine growth inexorably stretches
these ligaments, they refer pain from their
attachment sites in the characteristic patterns
of the following diagrams:

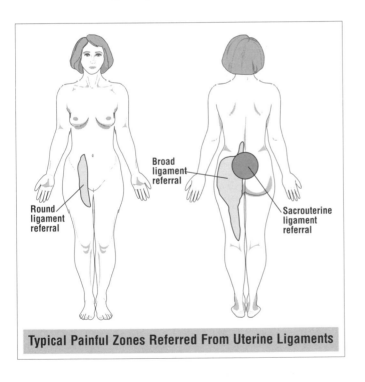

Typical Painful Zones Referred From Uterine Ligaments

♦ **Broad ligaments** — low
back, buttock, and sciatica-
like pain, especially in the
sixth month, and disap-
pearing in the seventh to
eighth months

♦ **Round ligaments** —
diagonal pain from top of
the uterus to groin; usually
one-sided, depending on
fetal position; sometimes as
extensive as the vulvar and
upper thigh fascia; more
common in the second
trimester

♦ **Sacrouterine ligaments** —
achiness just lateral to or
beneath the sacrum, espe-
cially in last trimester

Pain in one or both buttocks that radiates down the posterior leg is occasionally not referred from the broad ligament. Severe postural imbalance in the lumbar

spine and pelvis and/or chronic piriformis tension may entrap and compress the sciatic nerve. Sciatic nerve pain (sciatica) is usually characterized by a burning sensation, and may be accompanied by tingling, numbness, and weakness in the legs.

Other musculoskeletal pain in pregnancy

*M*any pregnant women complain of pain in the feet, legs, hips, and arms. Edema produces some of this achy, sore, tense feeling, as does strain to the muscles and joints of the feet and legs. Numbness around the medial malleolus and medial plantar aspect of the foot can occur if edema compresses the tibial nerve (tarsal tunnel syndrome), and the carpal tunnel can be similarily compromised. Cramping in both the gastrocnemius/soleus group and the peroneals torments some women's sleep, as does the vibration and irritated feeling of "restless legs." Compression of knee and ankle joints results in soreness and fatigue. Hip joint discomfort and stiffness caused by compression and chronic external rotation of the femur in the acetabulum often become more severe in later pregnancy when sleeping positions are restricted to sidelying or semireclining.[50]

Prior postural imbalances and injuries often exacerbated by pregnancy include lumbar and cervical lordosis, scoliosis, disc dysfunctions, and thoracic outlet syndrome. Thoracic outlet syndrome, with its characteristic pain, numbness, or tingling in the entire hand and along the arm, is intensified when the brachial plexus is further compressed by poor prenatal postural organization. Ribcage pain may occur as organ space diminishes in later pregnancy. The baby may intensify this discomfort with frequent kicks and strenuous stretching movements.

Headaches are often musculoskeletal in origin, referring from tension, strain, and trigger points, especially in the neck and upper back. They often increase in intensity and frequency with hyperventilation and hormonal effects on blood vessel dilation and increased mucous production in the sinuses.

> *"I came in with a splitting headache, but I could really feel my neck and shoulders relaxing in places that I didn't even know were tense. The visualization exercises helped too. I loved when she held the baby up for me and took the weight off my spine!"* — Susan

Massage therapy and pain control

*G*iven the far-ranging scope of these many structural changes, an expectant client's discomforts are understandable. Supporting and encouraging the body's adaptation to these myofascial and proprioceptive transitions is one of the key roles of the pre- and perinatal somatic practitioner. Massage therapy techniques are helpful in reducing muscle spasms, cramps, fibrosis, and other myofascial pain.[51]

Documentation of the effectiveness of massage therapy in reducing pain is relevant to maternity massage therapy practice. In one study, twice weekly massage therapy for four weeks significantly reduced physiological back and headache pain. Subjects benefited from a decrease in muscle tension, mental and physical strain, fatigue, and depression. They expressed a feeling of greater vitality and improved in mood and tension perception assessments.[52]

Fibromyalgia sufferers who received 30-minute sessions twice weekly for five weeks reported lower anxiety and depression, and their cortisol levels were lower immediately after sessions on the first and last days of the study. They also improved on objective measures of pain, reporting less fatigue and stiffness, and less sleep difficulty.[53]

The successful relief of pregnancy-related back pain reported by clients may be explained by the findings of the 1987 Quebec Task Force on Spinal Disorders. Their research suggested that massage reduces pain by alleviating painful stimulation and altering the processing of painful input. (See pain in labor, Chapter 4.) Massage also may affect the conduction of pain impulses in the peripheral nerves.[54]

> *"I was unable to sympathize with my pregnant friend's severe back pain because, fortunately, I learned ways to prevent backaches from my massage therapist. What pain I had was extremely mild and handled weekly in my sessions."* Jennifer

In his *Physician's Guide to Massage Therapy*, John Yates, Ph.D. theorizes that "kneading and stretching of the contracted muscle can be expected to elicit inhibitory reflex responses from tendon proprioceptors, which should contribute immediately to the relief of spasm. Also, improved circulation within the muscle as a result of massage should be directly beneficial by assisting in the removal of metabolic wastes and interrupting the 'pain-tension cycle' that involves ischemic pain."[55]

In taut, painfully spasmed muscles, selected muscle fibers can be relaxed with techniques that reset the muscle spindles and the Golgi tendon organs, such as strain and counterstrain[56] and other positional release techniques.

Pain-reducing methods that increase circulation of blood and lymph, such as Swedish massage and lymph drainage techniques, are appropriate pre- and peri-natally. Deep tissue work and other forms of myofascial release reduce pain by elongating shortened, bunched connective tissue.[57] Resisted movements, rhythmic passive movements (including small amplitude Trager® movements), and osteopathic strain and counterstrain and muscle energy techniques, are all effective in pain management.[58] Additionally, deep cross-fiber friction (Cyriax method) reduces pain and the restricted range of movement caused by fibrosis.[59]

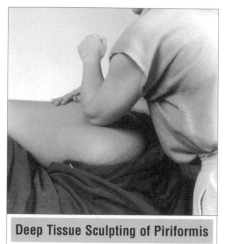

Deep Tissue Sculpting of Piriformis

Myofascial pain syndromes (trigger points), formerly known as myalgia, fibrositis, myositis, or rheumatism, are especially common for the woman coping with the structural stresses of pregnancy. These hyperirritable spots, described thoroughly by Dr. Janet Travell and Dr. David Simons,[60] usually occur within a taut band of skeletal muscle or in that muscle's fascia. They are quite painful when pressed, and they generally create a characteristic referred pain in some other location, sometimes very distant from the trigger point.

Trigger points, caused by trauma, poor posture, or by muscle chilling, fatigue, strain, or tension, are potential complaints of expectant mothers. Most prenatal trigger points develop in the musculature of the abdomen, ribcage, upper and lower back, neck, and legs. Focused pressure and massage over the trigger point, combined with appropriate stretching and other treatment options, have been shown to reduce the pain associated with these points by relieving tissue ischemia and allowing restoration of normal tissue blood supply.[61] (See abdominal precautions, Chapter 2.) The resulting reduction or elimination of neck and back pain experienced by many pregnant women brings welcome relief.

In addition to hands-on techniques, educational activities are effective interventions for reducing pain and decreasing stress on the weight-bearing joints and other myofascial structures. Correct and safe abdominal strengthening activities and body-use guidelines for walking, sitting, sleeping, carrying, and other daily activities will further reduce strain in the neck, back, and pelvis.[62] Introducing more efficient movement patterns enhances and reinforces the effectiveness of hands-on therapy, including those listed above for pain and spasm reduction.

LABOR PREPARATION

*P*hysical flexibility and kinesthetic awareness equip a woman to more actively participate in the birth process. Muscle and joint flexibility, particularly in the pelvis and legs, allows a laboring woman choices in birthing her baby. Pliable hip joints, supple adductors, hamstrings, and calf muscles, and resilient postural muscles respond positively to the urge of many laboring women to labor in a variety of positions.[63] At the very least, a woman birthing vaginally must be able to open her thighs to allow the baby's passage.

The same massage therapy methods useful for pain control are effective in increasing flexibility, especially passive and assisted-resisted stretching, deep tissue work, and the osteopathic soft-tissue treatments. Many women enjoy exercise and stretching, and find these activities to be safe, successful labor preparation, under the guidance of fitness or yoga instructors with specialized prenatal training.[64-67] Women should consult with their prenatal healthcare provider concerning the advisability of prenatal exercise.

Creating an awareness "bond" with her body is one of the many potential benefits of prenatal exercise and bodywork.[68] As a result of the "feedback loop" of the sensory-motor system, increased bodily awareness creates increased sensory awareness and muscle control.[69]

> "I believe that massage therapy helped me so much while I was pregnant. My body would relax, and I'd be so centered within myself and able to focus and go inside, which made a big difference during labor." — Andrea

This feedback loop is activated by the variety of stimuli introduced by body-work techniques. There are modulations in depth, direction, and duration of touch, especially in Swedish, deep tissue, and reflexive modalities. Kinesthetic input variations result from modifications in speed, rhythm, and intensity of passive and active movements, such as passive stretches, rhythmic passive movements (trepidations), assisted-resisted movements, and exercise. All of these experiences create a rich influx of information and corresponding responses and awareness in the client's body and mind. The result is heightened perception, new body understandings, and specifically localized awareness.

In order to give birth with less effort, the musculature of a woman's back, abdomen, and pelvic floor must remain relaxed to allow the uterus to labor without resistance. Relaxation of these muscles allows the baby to press more firmly against the cervix. The laboring woman must scan for and recognize tension throughout her body. She must know how, through imagery or conscious control, to release tension. Sometimes she must utilize specific muscles, such as the diaphragm, abdominals, or pelvic floor, in a precise, controlled manner. All of these abilities are developed in the process of receiving and responding to prenatal bodywork. Education in diaphragmatic breathing, pelvic floor strengthening (Kegel exercises), perineal self-massage, and abdominal strengthening are

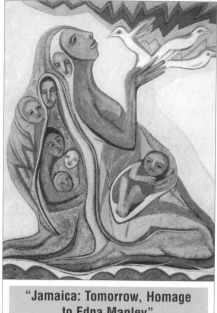

"Jamaica: Tomorrow, Homage to Edna Manley"
Acrylic painting by Betty La Duke
Used with artist's permission

particularly useful in developing awareness and control of these vital birthing muscles.[70]

Receiving therapeutic bodywork during pregnancy results in self-awareness, relaxation, and emotional support; they contribute to the development of a woman who is more able to access those inborn skills and intuitions that have evolved over the millennia of humanity's existence, activating what Nancy and Michael Samuels call the "three-million-year-old mother."[71]

LABOR FACILITATION

Massage therapy and other tactile support in labor

*R*esearch is verifying what many women inherently know: supportive, nurturing touch during labor can enhance emotional satisfaction, and diminish pain and the necessity for medical interventions. Several labor studies have reflected women's perception that "rubbing and massage" specifically improved their ability to cope with labor,[72] reduced labor pain,[73] met their emotional and physical needs, and provided relaxation.[74] The Touch Research Institute at the University of Miami conducted the most recent and specific study of massage for laboring women. Mothers receiving massage from their partners during labor experienced decreased levels of anxiety and pain. They needed less medication, and their labors were shorter than those of the control group receiving routine obstetrical care only.[75]

Massage therapy techniques are as effective during labor as they are prenatally. They reduce stress and promote relaxation; relieve muscle tension, cramping, and other soft-tissue discomforts; and support the physiological and emotional needs that naturally arise during labor and birth. As detailed in the previous section on stress in pregnancy and in the labor chapter to follow, stress reduces blood flow to the uterus by as much as 65% and contributes to long, slow, highly painful, unproductive labors. Relaxation facilitates labor and allows a woman to explore the many aspects of the labor process.

In a study of touch during active labor, nurses provided laboring women a high degree of nurturing and reassuring contact, such as stroking the brow and hand holding, in addition to the clinical necessities of pulse taking and cervical exams. After three contractions, they then offered only clinical touch for three contractions. During the three contractions of high contact, pulse rate and systolic blood pressure dropped, and women appeared to be more comfortably coping with their labors than at other times.[76]

These studies validate the value of touch inherent in the work of those providing professional labor support. Extensive studies of their work has been conducted by John Kennell, M.D., Marshall Klaus, M.D., Phyllis Klaus, Ph.D., and Ellen Hodnett.[77, 78, 79] Also known as "doulas," labor support professionals are women whose role is to provide physical and emotional support throughout labor. A doula typically spends most of her time stroking, kneading, holding, and physically and/or verbally comforting her charge. In a meta-analysis of six of Kennell and

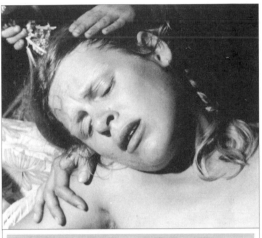

Skillful, Comforting Touch Eases Labor Pain
Photograph used by permission of Harriette Hartigan

Klaus's studies, this consistent physical presence, nurturing touch, and emotional support created the following benefits for the experimental group compared to the control groups:

- 25% shorter labor times
- 40% less use of oxytocin (labor stimulant)
- 30% decrease in all pain medication use, including 60% decrease in requests for epidurals
- 40% less need for forceps
- 50% fewer cesarean births
- Improved infant Apgar scores
- Enhanced familial social adjustment postpartum[80]

Though studies have yet to be focused on the effects of a highly-trained somatic practitioner on labor outcomes, results comparable to the doula studies seem likely. Meanwhile, innumerable, detailed anecdotal evidence of these benefits is accumulating in the professional records of prenatal massage therapists and other somatic practitioners.

"Delivery on my due date was particularly important to me as I was trying to avoid a c-section if I was past due. I believe that learning to use

the pressure points contributed to a safe, on-time birth, in addition to labor pain relief. I'll definitely have massage therapy with my next baby, too." — Carrie

"We wanted a gentle, unmedicated birth, but six hours of intense labor almost ended in a cesarean. My therapist used every massage technique to keep my hips relaxed and pressed on them. Then she cradled me on my side to help the baby come out." — Pat

The long-term value of appropriate labor massage therapy is undeniable. More women express satisfaction with their childbirth experience and its impact on their lives when they are emotionally supported during labor. In fact, nurturing care correlates more significantly with this satisfaction than with the ease of the physical process of labor, even in long, complicated births.[81, 82]

Encouraging Nurturing Maternal Touch

*P*renatal massage therapy provides women with an experience of nurturing, respectful touch; an experience often lacking in the technological, touch-aversive atmosphere of many Western cultures. Negative developmental impacts, including neglect, impersonal physical contact, and physical, sexual, and emotional abuse, further deprive some women of an embodied sense of appropriate, loving touch.

The impact of touch deprivation is not simply a matter of reduced sensory pleasures and optional physical indulgences. Sociological research of American orphanages of the early 1900s noted a 95% to 100% mortality rate for infants with only institutional care and little or no tactile and/or vestibular stimulation.[83] More recently, widespread media coverage publicized the developmental tragedies of deprived children neglected in communist-regime Romanian orphanages.[84]

Animal studies have clearly demonstrated the deleterious physical and emotional effects of tactile deprivation. Mice that were handled during their infancy nursed, cleaned, and cared for their young better than those in unstroked control groups.[85] Many of Harry Harlow's test monkeys who were separated from their mothers became depressed and violent, and repeated autistic, withdrawn, and stimulus seeking behaviors such as rocking, head banging, and sucking.[86] Brain function of several of the most severely affected monkeys were subsequently studied, revealing abnormal electrophysiological discharges when compared to the brains of normal monkeys.[87]

James Prescott, Ph.D., neuropsychologist and former head of the Developmental Behavioral Biology Program at the National Institute of Health, theorizes from studying Harlow's monkeys that during formative periods of brain growth, lack of sensory input of normal touching and rocking by the mother damages the development of the neuronal systems that control affection. These individuals are less capable of love and pleasure and more inclined toward violence, depression, and isolation. Prescott extended his study of the origins of love and violence, correlating cultural anthropologists' data on infant physical affection and adult physical violence. His final conclusions showed a 73% correlation in forty-nine societies between high infant physical attention, including caressing and carrying the infant on the mother's body, and low crime and violence, including theft, torture, mutilation, and slavery.[88]

> *"I learned so much in my massages about appropriate levels of touch and so many techniques I can utilize to get in touch with my baby in the womb, and after she's born."* — Sara

Massage practitioners have the opportunity to positively impact their clients' and humanity's nurturing skills. They can become role models from whom their pregnant clients learn loving, appropriate touch. This potential is best illustrated by the work of nursing professor and researcher, Reva Rubin, R.N. Rubin conducted many observational studies on maternal behaviors during her career at the University of Pittsburgh Nursing School.[89, 90] Using behavioral rating scales, she noted that both first-time and experienced mothers progressed similarly in touching their newborns. Initial touch was with tentative fingertips, then fuller hand contact, and finally complete arm embraces, leading to "molding" of the two to each other. This sequence appeared to be completed more slowly, or to be interrupted or aborted, by those women whose prenatal and perinatal care consisted only of routine, impersonal medical touch. She concluded that "appropriate, meaningful touch of pregnant and laboring women leads to touching babies in meaningful, effective, and caring ways," thus facilitating the transformation of a daughter into a mother.[91]

Additionally, massage practitioners may teach women and their partners selective prenatal, labor, and/or infant massage techniques. While therapeutic procedures requiring refined palpatory skills and advanced anatomical knowledge are inappropriate to teach to lay people, non-professionals may safely stroke and knead family members when important safety precautions are included in instruction. Prenatal and labor massage instruction prepares and empowers partners and other loved ones to offer meaningful physical nurturing to the mother.

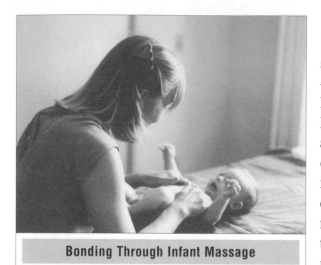

Bonding Through Infant Massage

Premature infants who received a 15-minute massage and movement sequence three times daily gained 47% more weight, secreted higher levels of cortisol and human growth hormones, and were more active, alert, and relaxed than unmassaged control preemies. They went home from the hospital an average of six days earlier, and these babies' superior development continued through the six months of follow-up study, regardless of whether the massage was continued at home.[92] This study, and numerous others [93-102] support the benefits of massage for infants and their caretakers, and make a convincing case for including infant massage instruction in pre- and perinatal massage therapy practices.[103]

POSTPARTUM RECOVERY

After childbirth, many women have an intrinsic need to recount the details of their experience. Some women retell their stories repeatedly, oftentimes unsolicited by family and friends. This storytelling can seem most urgent for those for whom the outcome of labor and birth was not as anticipated, or for whom there was a significant feeling of loss of control. The psychological repercussions of childbearing profoundly influence more than the mother; each individual family member, friends, and other associates are affected. The psychological integration of her childbearing experience is a critical aspect of postpartum recovery.[104]

"I had two miscarriages prior to receiving bodywork. Through the course of my sessions, I discovered a lot of stored-up feelings regarding a child I'd carried and delivered many years prior to these losses. I was able to process my feelings regarding that baby and the feelings around the miscarriages. My next pregnancy produced my precious Brittany."
— Lindsey

Massage practitioners provide a professional yet caring opportunity for postpartum women to share their experiences. Within a therapeutic session, many women will want to celebrate their accomplishments and to unburden themselves of the fear, sadness, and anger often generated during labor. Recounting trying moments, frightening interventions, and frustrations with the process, they can begin to let go of muscular tension, frozen expressions and gestures, and unresolved issues.

In addition to providing emotional support, the somatic practitioner facilitates physiological recovery of the exhausted postpartum woman. Circulatory, deep tissue, trigger point, and other reflexive massage methods help to cleanse lactic acid and medication residues from tissues, reduce muscle strain, and clear any soft-tissue dysfunction generated in the athleticism of labor. Physiological assistance is especially helpful for post-cesarean mothers who are recuperating from major abdominal surgery, as well as the strain of pregnancy. Appropriate, sequential therapy to the incision site may speed healing and reduce fibrous buildup in and around the scar.[105]

> *"After my c-section I came in a week later to get a massage. My recovery was quicker than my previous two c-sections. Scar tissue was minimized by the massage work that was done to the incision. It was also a great support to me to have someone to confide in as far as the nursing."* — Maria

Constipation, difficulty urinating, uterine cramping, and perineal soreness are common in the days and weeks postpartum. Skin rolling, trigger point therapy, and Swedish abdominal techniques reduce these pains and aid rehabilitation of the abdominal skin, muscles, and organs.[106] Reflexive techniques to feet, hands, connective tissue, and energy meridians may enhance metabolic functioning, systemically and in individual organs.[107] Practitioners may help women recognize the extent of any diastus recti and guide them toward progressive, appropriate toning exercises.[108]

Many postpartum women continue to experience pain from pregnancy postural imbalances that may have been exacerbated while laboring. Further structural stresses occur during the many hours of nursing, bending, lifting, carrying, and playing required by childcare. The practitioner offers relief from postural and mechanically-induced postpartum pain by reducing tension in postural muscles; reeducating the mother about the use of the iliopsoas muscles for both pelvic alignment and efficient gait; and encouraging proper body mechanics.

Summary of benefits

*P*arents, maternity healthcare providers, and somatic practitioners can feel confident and enthused about the contributions that skilled, empathetic touch therapies make to individual women, their families, and the human family. Pre- and perinatal massage therapy offers far-reaching, multi-dimensional beneficial influences.

Benefits of Massage Therapy

During Pregnancy

- Reduces stress, promotes relaxation, facilitates transitions through emotional support and physical nurturing
- Reduces edema and blood pressure, relieves varicose veins, and increases blood and lymph circulation
- Facilitates hormonal, respiratory, gastrointestinal, urinary, and other physiological processes during pregnancy
- Reduces musculoskeletal strain and pain
- Contributes to developing flexibility and the kinesthetic awareness necessary to actively participate in the birth process
- Fosters nurturing maternal touch

In Labor

- Contributes to shorter, less painful labor
- Reduces labor complications, medications, and interventions
- Improves infant well-being

In the Postpartum Period

- Facilitates postpartum emotional, physiological, and family adjustments
- Reduces musculoskeletal and organic pain
- Promotes structural realignment of the spine and pelvis, and reorganization of movement
- Contributes to rehabilitation of abdominal skin, muscles, and organs
- Promotes recovery from cesarean birth, including healing of the incision
- Relieves muscle strain caused by childcare activities

In Society

- Develops individuals more capable of love and pleasure
- Builds less violent, more respectful cultures

Chapter

2

Guidelines and Precautions for Prenatal Massage Therapy

*P*re- and perinatal massage therapy is not intended to replace prenatal care by physicians, nurse-midwives, and midwives. These professionals ensure vital monitoring of gestational progress and maternal health. As adjunctive providers, somatic practitioners are more effective when working in collaboration with a woman's healthcare provider.

Whether in independent practice or under direct medical supervision, practitioners must understand the clinical applications of pregnancy physiology including: positioning, depth of pressure, safety precautions, contraindications, technique modifications, prenatal complications, and high-risk factors.

POSITIONING CONCERNS

*T*he question most practitioners initially consider when contemplating massaging pregnant women is positioning: "How will I accommodate that ripe belly?" When accustomed to the supine and prone positions, both practitioner and client often feel limited to these options. Many practitioners are especially stumped by the dilemma of how to massage an aching back crying out for care, other than with the client in the prone (face down) position.

There are several relevant issues involved in this practical dilemma. The safety of the mother and the baby is of utmost concern to both the client and the practitioner. Establishing secure positions that will neutralize or reduce strain to soft tissues is another priority. Pregnant clients will not appreciate massage therapy received in positions that strain areas already impacted by postural and physiological stresses. The prone position is particularly problematic in all of these regards.

Prone positioning restrictions

*S*ome women like to sleep on their belly or in a ¾ prone position with pillow supports through much of their pregnancy. This may be a safe, comfortable resting position, but once pressure is applied for massage this is no longer a reliably safe option. Prone positioning on a flat therapy table exerts strain on the lumbar, pelvic, and uterine structures. Posterior musculature is shortened; the lumbar vertebra and lumbosacral junction are compressed and anteriorly displaced; the sacroiliac joints are rotated; and strain on the sacrouterine ligaments is increased. Obviously, the prone position aggravates the very causes of many women's back discomfort, particularly in later pregnancy.

Some practitioners may attempt to accommodate the pregnant belly and mechanically reduce lumbar strain by placing pillows under the chest and pelvic regions, by propping the upper torso on a stack of pillows, or by using equipment that is marketed as "the solution" for prone positioning for pregnant women. Neither pillow props, body cushions, pregnancy pillows, most on-site massage chairs, nor tables with cut-out ovals, with or without a sling or net designed to support the belly, solves the problematic aspects of prone positioning. These alternatives either (1) further strain the taxed uterine ligaments, especially the sacrouterine ligaments, by dangling the uterus from these attachments, or (2) create increased intrauterine pressure, particularly when sufficient pressure is applied to therapeutically address the posterior structures.

Increased intrauterine pressure is probably not a significant safety concern in the first trimester, or in most normal, uncomplicated, low-risk pregnancies. It is of particular relevance when there are abnormalities in placental attachment or function, or a higher risk of such conditions. More caution is also prudent if there is concern about fetal blood supply or uterine competence. Women who have been diagnosed with these conditions are often uninformed about their impact with regard to receiving massage therapy. Some of these problems go undetected until

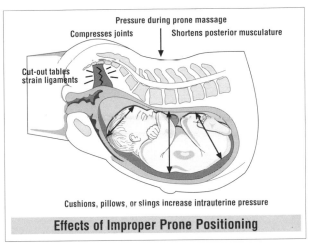

Pressure during prone massage
Compresses joints   Shortens posterior musculature

Cut-out tables strain ligaments

Cushions, pillows, or slings increase intrauterine pressure

Effects of Improper Prone Positioning

bleeding, cramping, or other overt signs of problems have occurred to warrant further diagnosis. If "doing no harm" is of highest priority, then the risk of excessive intrauterine pressure must be avoided with all pregnant clients.

Prone positioning involves the additional discomfort of pressure on breasts that are often very tender and sensitive, even in the first trimester when the abdomen is not significantly larger. Because of increased mucous production and the inability to use antihistamines and other allergy and sinus medications, many women become unacceptably congested in prone position as well. Some women are both uneasy and uncomfortable with the concept of "lying on their baby," and they find settling into a receptive prone position impossible. Finally, to complete the argument against prone pregnancy positioning, verbal and emotional sharing is hampered for many by the confines of face cradles and other devices which position the head when lying face down.

For the comfort and safety of the pregnant woman, eliminate the prone position after the first 13 weeks, regardless of the client's perception or preferences in this regard. Modify prenatal techniques usually performed with the client prone to other, safer positions.

Supine positioning guidelines

Supine positioning also involves safety considerations in pregnancy. In this position the weighty uterus rests against the inferior vena cava. The major vessel of blood return to the heart, the vena cava runs up the right sides of the vertebral bodies along the posterior abdominal wall. Extended compression of the vena cava will result in low maternal blood pressure and decreased circulation both to the mother and her baby (supine hypotensive syndrome). After five or more minutes, some women report uneasiness, dizziness, shortness of breath, or other discomforts when lying flat on their backs, although others seem entirely content.[1] With or without notable negative effects, however, decreased fetal circulation occurs, particularly if the placenta is embedded posteriorly.

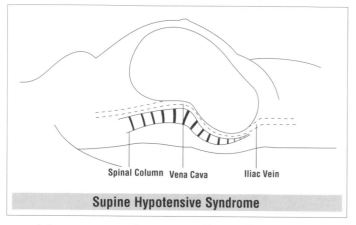

Supine Hypotensive Syndrome

Spinal Column   Vena Cava   Iliac Vein

The American College of Obstetricians and Gynecologists (ACOG), generally regarded as the ranking U.S. authority in obstetrical policies, cautions women against vigorous exercise in supine position after four months (22 weeks).[2] With these recommendations, it would appear safe for women receiving massage therapy to lie on their backs briefly (two to five minute maximum after 13 weeks) throughout pregnancy. In second and third trimesters, however, mitigating measures for more extended supine positioning are prudent. Options for decreasing obstruction of the vena cava in the second trimester include use of pillow support under the right side of the torso to shift uterine weight toward the left. After 22 weeks, elevate the torso to a semireclined angle. (See specific requirements of these alterations, Chapter 3.) Adapt prenatal techniques usually performed with the client supine for these positions. Some women are advised by their healthcare provider to never lie flat on their backs, primarily when there is increased concern about fetal oxygenation. Always observe these instructions, regardless of your or your client's perception or preferences in this regard.

The supine position can aggravate the sacroiliac (SI) joints and cause back pain, especially if the back is poorly supported, or on an inadequately padded table, or the woman is in the last trimester. Supine positioning can create an immediate, painful, locking sensation in the upper buttock and iliac crest, usually on one side. This is caused by imbalance and strain to the sacroiliac joints, particularly if one SI joint is hypomobile and the other is hypermobile.[3] Since hard surfaces are more problematic than soft ones, two and one half inches of triple density foam padding is a minimum requirement on massage therapy tables. For client comfort and safety, always support and reduce lumbar lordosis with a Contoured bodyCushion® (see Resources appendix) or a small lumbar pillow, and sufficient knee bolsters.

Sidelying positioning

*T*he discussions of the prone and supine positions in pregnancy begin to substantiate a protocol for prenatal massage therapy that recognizes the superiority of the sidelying (lateral recumbent) position for maximum safety and comfort throughout all pregnancies. The sidelying position prevents increased sinus pressure and tends to encourage somatoemotional integration. When sufficiently supported by pillows, bolsters, and or cushions, **most** women find maximum comfort in the sidelying position. Strain on any of the uterine

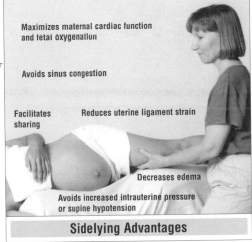

Maximizes maternal cardiac function and fetal oxygenation

Avoids sinus congestion

Facilitates sharing

Reduces uterine ligament strain

Decreases edema

Avoids increased intrauterine pressure or supine hypotension

Sidelying Advantages

ligaments or on the musculoskeletal structures is minimized. Dangerously increased intrauterine pressure is avoided. (See specific requirements for creating sufficient support, Chapter 3.) In fact, the sidelying position is **recommended** by physicians and midwives when addressing placental and fetal circulation concerns. The left sidelying position allows maximum maternal cardiac functioning and fetal oxygenation.[4] Again, with a primary commitment to "first do no harm," the safest position for prenatal massage therapy is the sidelying position, regardless of possible inconvenience to or preference of the practitioner.

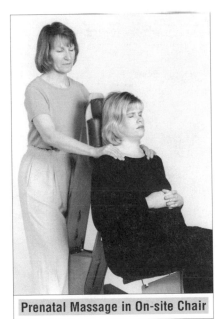

Prenatal Massage in On-site Chair

Another safe option, although generally not as comfortable for the expectant client, is seated massage therapy. When using a chair or stool, choose one that allows maximum access to the client and that is comfortable without being overly soft. On-site massage chairs are a safe alternative only when the pregnant client semi-reclines against the pad normally utilized for chest support, for the same reasons as described in the prone positioning discussion above.

Positioning Guidelines Summary

First Trimester

♦ Supine, prone, sidelying, semireclining, or in a chair, depending on client comfort

♦ Adjust for breast tenderness

Second Trimester

♦ Prone position is not recommended, even with specialized equipment such as "cut-out" tables or cushions

♦ Supine - use pillow under right lower torso, up to week 22. After week 22, supine is not recommended; use semireclining and sidelying positions only to prevent supine hypotensive syndrome; chair okay

Third Trimester

♦ Sidelying and semireclining positions only; chair okay

DEPTH OF PRESSURE/PAIN LEVEL

"I loved my first experience with massage therapy. I definitely feared it would be too harsh; it was nothing like that. It was warm, attentive, and wonderful. I wished it would go on forever. I felt more balanced, and the specific tight areas I had just melted." — Roselle

*I*f positioning is the practitioner's first concern, generally the second is appropriate pressure and pain levels: "Pregnant women seem so vulnerable, yet I've been trained to work very deeply in order for the work to work." With maternity massage, always ascertain the client's pressure preferences, perception of pain, tension level, and needs in a given body area. Her general health, injuries, and other safety considerations discussed later in this chapter often dictate lighter pressures.

Providing her with a reliable means to express her experience, such as a number or color-coded scale, allows her to communicate beyond generalized responses such as "that feels okay." Some practitioners are successful with a number scale method of labeling pain level. Probably the most frequently used is:

0	Pressure only
1 - 5	Pressure perceived as pleasurable
5.5 - 7	Increasing pressure is beginning to change from purely pleasurable into mild discomfort; however, that discomfort still feels good
7.5 - 10	More pain than pleasure, becoming intolerable at 10

Many women relate well to a color scheme for pleasure/pain feedback that follows the common correlation of a traffic light:

Green	Completely pleasurable	Keep on going
Yellow	Pleasure tinged with mild discomfort to mild pain, but still feels good	Proceed with caution
Red	More pain than pleasure	Stop

Maintaining an awareness of the pleasure/pain level also assures that neither the mother nor the fetus is stimulated to sympathetic arousal. Pain activates adrenal production of the hormones which elevate blood pressure, heart rate, and respiratory rate and which lower immune function and blood flow to the uterus. Since these hormonal signals diffuse into fetal circulation through the placenta, the fetus is similarly negatively impacted.[5]

Forceful and abrupt movements also activate the client's defensive withdrawal reflexes that trigger increased muscular tension rather than relaxation. At high pain levels, the crossed extensor reflex activates the extensors of the opposite limb and may cause the entire body to push away from the source of pain. Remember, it is only in a receptive state that new behaviors, such as correct breathing, relaxation, and postural alignment are readily and thoroughly explored and learned.[6] If the pregnant client is to realize the benefits of somatic therapies, then perform even the deepest work gently.

EFFECTIVE PRE- AND PERINATAL SOMATIC THERAPIES

*M*any effective touch therapies are adaptable for maternity care. Promoting any one method or procedural sequence as the maternity massage therapy would deprive women of the wide-ranging benefits of the many somatic practices available to the professional massage practitioner. While later chapters include instruction in a number of essential techniques, seek reliable hands-on education in several or all of the methodologies described below so that you may address the multidimensional needs of childbearing women. To ensure complete, accurate information, always consult master teachers of a particular method for reliable pre- and perinatal information. This is particularly important in the case of the eastern reflexive techniques, such as acupressure and shiatsu, as these methods are only overviewed in this text.

During the childbearing year, specific techniques often must be significantly modified and others eliminated. Use this text's guidelines and this chapter's precautions to carefully evaluate the physiological, structural, and psychological impact of every technique from any method contemplated for pregnancy, labor, and postpartum use. Complete a comprehensive educational program, such as the "Pre- and Perinatal Massage Therapy" certification workshop, for demonstrations and hands-on practice of specifically adapted, effective techniques.[7]

<u>Assisted-Resisted Stretches</u>: Practitioner-directed movement by client is resisted by practitioner to activate stretch receptors in the muscles and joints and facilitate muscular relaxation; similar to proprioceptive neuromuscular facilitation (PNF) or muscle energy techniques.[8]

<u>Aston-Patterning</u>®: Education in movement, ergonomics, and fitness, in conjunction with bodywork techniques designed for each individual to facilitate optimal expression and function. Created by Judith Aston.

<u>Craniosacral Therapy</u>: Method of evaluating and enhancing the function of the craniosacral system, including the brain, spinal cord, and related fascial structures using a variety of gentle pressures, tractions, and positioning techniques; created by Andrew T. Still, D.O., and developed by John E. Upledger, D.O.[9]

<u>Cross-Fiber Friction (Deep Compression Massage)</u>: Deep pressure with thumb or fingers across the axis of the muscle fiber, across specific lesions in muscle bellies, musculotendinous junctions, tendons, teno-periosteal junctions, or ligaments; created by James Cyriax, M.D.[10]

<u>Deep Tissue Massage (Myofascial Release)</u>: Slow, specific strokes with thumbs, fingers, or elbows through fascial planes and muscles to release habitual patterns of holding in myofascial tissue.

Deep tissue sculpting: Deep tissue massage using hands, elbows, or fingertips, to slowly melt or stroke through contractions in fascia or muscles along the axis of muscle fiber and usually from muscle origin to insertion; proceeds only at speed of release of tissue, and not beyond pleasure/pain intensity; developed by Carole Osborne-Sheets.[11]

Structural balancing: Deep compressions and strokes through fascial planes usually executed simultaneously with directed, active movements by the client; intended to reeducate movement, organize fascia, and balance structure; based on the principles of Ida P. Rolf, Ph.D., and developed by Edward Maupin, Ph.D. and others.[12, 13]

Skin Rolling: Deep tissue massage movement using fingertips and thumbs of both hands to lift and loosen a section of skin, superficial fascia, and underlying deep fascia.[14]

<u>Lomi-Lomi</u>: Hawaiian technique using thumbs to perform moving, cross-fiber friction across the axis of a muscle belly; developed by Margaret Machado.[15]

<u>Lymphatic Drainage</u>: Circulatory movement using fingertips or flat of palm to create suction effect in lymphatic channels of skin, superficial fascia, or muscles.[16]

<u>Passive Movements</u>: Practitioner performs movements of varying amplitude, intensity, and speed that gently move the body or move specific joints.[17, 18]

Blends (also deep tissue/passive movement blends): Use of both deep tissue and passive movement techniques, performed simultaneously; usually one hand creates motion while other sculpts myofascial tension; created by Carole Osborne-Sheets.[19, 20]

Joint Mobilization: Movement of joint through range of motion until barrier (rubbery end feel) to motion is felt. Joint is then held in position of ease (away from barrier).

Rhythmic Passive Movements (Trepidations): Small amplitude and continuous rhythmic movements that are intended to induce relaxation of muscles habitually tensed and to increase quality and quantity of movement.[21]

Strain and Counterstrain (Positional release, "fold and hold"): Relief of "tender points" in soft tissues by positioning client in maximal comfort position and holding for 90 seconds; created by Lawrence Jones, D.O.[22, 23]

Stretching: Mechanical tension applied to lengthen the myofascial unit (muscles and fascia). Longitudinal and cross-directional are two types of stretching.[24]

Traction: Use of therapist's body weight to create a gradual, gentle tensile pull on a specific joint or body area to reduce compression of joints and tension in surrounding soft tissue.

Reflex Massage: Massage techniques directed to cutaneous or neurological referral zones for the purpose of effecting either systemic change or local change at distant "referred" sites. Techniques may vary from light to very deep digital pressure.

Acupressure (Shiatsu): Use of fingers to apply deep pressure to specific points on the body that are effective in promoting balanced flow of vital energy through specific acupuncture pathways (meridians).[25]

Connective tissue massage (*Bindegewebsmassage*): Reflex stroke using the tips of finger or fingers to drag and pull through skin and/or superficial fascia along specific dermatomes to activate parasympathetic arousal and increase vascularization of area; German medical massage method created by Elizabeth Dicke.[26]

Reflexology (Zone Therapy): Reflex massage of the feet using thumbs or fingertips to compress undifferentiated nerves in the skin against bone at specific sites to create a distant effect; also performed on hands; developed by Ina Bryant and Eunice Ingham.[27]

Trigger Point Massage (Neuromuscular Therapy): Deep ischemic compression of individual areas of hypersensitivity in muscles, ligaments, tendons, and fascia, called trigger points. These trigger points are defined by their local tenderness and referral of pain to distant locations in muscles, connective tissue, and organs; originated by Janet Travell, M. D. and David Simons, M.D.; developed by Bonnie Prudden, Paul St. John, Judith Walker Delaney, and others.[28]

Somatoemotional Integration: Use of soft tissue techniques, movement, and verbal exploration to reduce tissue dysfunction, mobilize the breath, and process emotional states which may be held in the physical frame; developed by Carole Osborne-Sheets.[29]

Swedish Massage (Circulatory): Traditional European massage which employs a variety of pushing, pulling, lifting, percussive, and compressing strokes to affect the underlying muscular and vascular systems; also employs "gymnastic" passive movements; may be performed very slowly and softly (Esalen style).[30, 31]

METHODOLOGICAL PRECAUTIONS AND CONTRAINDICATIONS

Abdominal massage

*M*iscarriage (spontaneous abortion) is a natural termination of pregnancy before the fetus has reached viability, generally before 20 weeks gestation and weighing less than 350 grams. Miscarriage occurs in some 15% of identified pregnancies, and early miscarriages before pregnancy is confirmed probably bring the total rate of miscarriage closer to 40% of conceptions.[32]

Preterm labor jeopardizes the health and lives of the mother and baby in 8% to 10% of pregnancies. Preterm labor involves regular contractions that dilate the cervix after 20 weeks and before the end of 36 weeks gestation. It is encouraging that technological advances have made the viability of these babies possible as early as 24 weeks; however, preemies' early weeks and months are fraught with risk. Many are born to teenage mothers, or into the challenges of poverty, drug abuse, and alcohol addiction.[33]

The death or injury of a baby, even the tiniest zygote, is a multifaceted issue for different individuals. Perhaps the most fundamental issue is one of loss — the loss of the child, a desired relationship, part of one's self, and of one's dreams. Most grieving parents seek to make sense of their tragedy, and they long to understand why and how this death occurred. Others involved in their care frequently suffer with them. In as many as half of pregnancy losses, injuries, and premature labors, the exact cause of problems is unknown.

Certain maternal conditions, high-risk factors, and complications of pregnancy may increase the occurrence of miscarriage or premature labor, including:

♦ Previous miscarriage or preterm labor
♦ Altered nutrition leading to low maternal weight gain
♦ Smoking and alcohol use, and exposure to other substances or environmental factors that cause fetal malformation such as radiation, chemicals, and other teratogens
♦ Drug abuse, especially cocaine
♦ Emotional stress
♦ Heavy work load at home or on the job
♦ Decreased blood flow to the uterus caused by:
  placenta abrupto, placenta previa, diabetes, renal disease, cardiovascular disease, systemic lupus and other autoimmune factors, preeclampsia, overdistension of the uterus in multiple gestations, and excess amniotic fluid (polyhydramnios)
♦ Abdominal trauma or surgery

- Premature rupture of membranes
- Diethylstilbestrol (DES) exposure in utero resulting in uterine abnormalities
- Incompetent cervix and other uterine anomalies
- Infection of the urinary tract, or vaginal or uterine diseases such as endometriosis
- Fever, and infectious diseases such as rubella, cytomegalovirus, active genital herpes, or toxoplasmosis
- Maternal age over 35
- Chromosomal abnormalities
- Extreme hypothermia[34]

One of the most common symptoms of premature labor and miscarriage is low back, thigh, and/or pelvic pain, referred from the contracting uterus; however, there are **usually** other identifying symptoms, such as bleeding, amniotic fluid leakage, abdominal cramping, or regular uterine contractions. (See complications below.) Ask the client's physician to rule out miscarriage, labor, or other possible causes of back pain, such as urinary tract infection, neurological dysfunctions, or prior, unresolved injuries before beginning or continuing massage therapy. Remember that musculoskeletal back pain is **usually** relieved with a client's change in position or activity, while referred organic pain is not. Take full prenatal and medical histories, and evaluate your client's progress thoroughly at each massage therapy session.

Never increase intrauterine pressure, decrease uterine blood flow, or press deeply or pointedly into the abdomen. Take these precautions to ensure the safety of the mother and her baby.

- Effectively position and support the pregnant client as detailed in Positioning section, in Chapter Three.
- Never perform any touch to the pregnant abdomen deeper than the skin and superficial fascia level or with pointed pressure (including the lateral abdomen, anterior of the quadratus lumborum, as well as those directly on the belly). While the effect of deep abdominal massage techniques on pregnancy has never been specifically

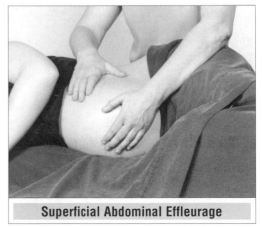

Superficial Abdominal Effleurage

studied, light, full-handed pressure avoids any possibility of abdominal trauma that may provoke uterine contractions or injure vulnerable structures. This precaution applies to any method of somatic practices including deep tissue, trigger point, and acupressure.

♦ Secure the client's permission before touching her abdomen. Some women prefer to skip abdominal techniques entirely or to learn techniques that they or their partners enjoy sharing with their baby. Strictly adhere to clients', midwives', and physicians' restrictions regarding abdominal massage. To ensure that neither they nor their clients would ever question the safety of their work, some practitioners prefer to entirely avoid touching a first trimester abdomen or the abdomen of those whose risk of miscarriage or preterm labor is high. (See list above and sections later in this chapter on complications and high-risk factors.)

> *"Regardless of the fact that I had uterine abnormalities, my doctor had no concerns that massage therapy would in any way interfere. Not only did the massage not interfere, it was tremendous physical and emotional support during this pregnancy with its threats of delivering early or mis-carrying altogether. It was very helpful to go to my therapist, not only for the reduction in stress, but also for the emotional support that I was given. It was very important to stay relaxed and calm through this preg-nancy, for the baby as well as myself."* — Jennifer

Circulatory system and massage therapy precautions

During pregnancy, the blood's clotting capacity increases to four or five times higher than non-pregnant levels. Because the **clot-dissolving** capacity (fibinolysis) decreases dramatically, women are more protected from potential hemorrhaging during childbirth; however, they also are more likely to develop blood clots (thrombi).[35] Thrombi are also the result of the growing gravid uterus restricting iliac and femoral circulation and contributing to sluggish blood flow; higher progesterone levels relaxing vascular smooth muscles; and increased metabolic demands elevating blood and interstitial fluid volumes.

Thrombosis can occur in any vein during pregnancy; however, clot formation is greatest in the veins where blood is most stagnant. The veins most likely to harbor clots during pregnancy are the deeper iliac, femoral, and saphenous veins.[36] When clots accumulate in these vessels, they may create some discom-fort, but they pose no major threat, unless inflammation and/or infection (throm-bophlebitis) develops. Deep vein thrombosis is more serious when clots dislodge, move into circulation, and occlude smaller vessels in the lungs (pulmonary embolism), heart (coronary thrombosis), or brain (cerebral embolism). These types of thromboembolisms occur five to six times more frequently in pregnancy.[37]

While most women will develop clots, the more sedentary a woman is, the higher the likelihood of thrombi. Women on bed rest are especially prone to clot production,[38] as are women over 30, those who are obese, have lupus, or are expecting their fourth or more baby.[39] Abruption of the placenta, preeclampsia/eclampsia, and intrauterine fetal death all increase clot formation, sometimes leading to a further serious complication involving generalized activation of the coagulation process (disseminated intravascular coagulaopathy).[40]

The characteristic symptoms of leg thrombi include increased edema in the foot and/or leg, localized swelling, heat, redness, and painful, achy legs. While these symptoms may indicate the presence of thrombi, swollen and achy legs unrelated to thrombosis are common in pregnancy. A clear determination of the presence of clots is also difficult because often thrombi are asymptomatic.[41]

Given the hypercoaguable state of pregnancy and potential harm of freely circulating clots, eliminate procedures which have the potential to flush thrombi from their likely harbors. Follow these guidelines.

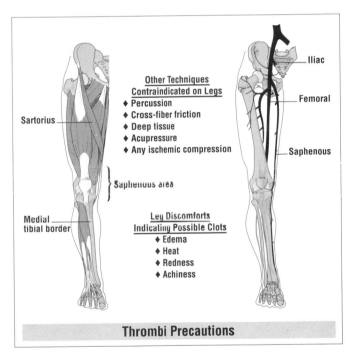

Thrombi Precautions

- ◆ Do not press deeply into the abdomen, especially in the inguinal area.
- ◆ Use only superficial, whole-hand pressure throughout the medial surface of the legs where problematic veins traverse, specifically along and posterior to the sartorius muscles, distal to the medial knees, and along the medial tibial borders.
- ◆ Perform no deep, pointed, or stationary pressure sufficiently sustained to restrict localized blood flow (ischemic pressure) in these areas, regardless of the type of technique and its otherwise potential benefits.
- ◆ Eliminate tapotement (percussion) from Swedish leg work, and limit cross-fiber friction, trigger point therapy, deep tissue, acupressure, and any other deep pressure to other, safer body parts.

♦ Eliminate leg work entirely when client is on bed rest, or if placental abruption, preeclampsia, reduced fetal movement, or other conditions increasing clot risks occur.

Following these guidelines will also protect vascular areas weakened by the hormonal effects of progesterone, including spider veins and varicose veins. Varicose veins and clots are most frequently found in the same blood vessels. In any areas of varicose or spider veins, additionally modify massage therapy techniques according to the severity of the condition:

<u>Mild</u>   (visible, convoluted, ropy veins): use only appropriate Swedish and lymphatic drainage strokes at moderate pressure

<u>Moderate</u> (palpable veins with convoluted pathways): appropriate Swedish and lymphatic drainage strokes using a light pressure

<u>Severe</u>   (palpable, raised veins, purplish, bruised surrounding tissue): use only featherlight touch; use other procedures that help relieve pelvic congestion

Reflexive techniques

*R*eflexology to the feet and hands stimulates relaxation, facilitates metabolic functions that support pregnancy, and helps to reduce common prenatal discomforts. Several reflexive areas require specific precautions during pregnancy, however.

Much anecdotal evidence indicates that deep, bone-to-bone pressure to the uterus and ovary zones can readily initiate labor or kick-start languid labor contractions. Obviously, then, any ishemic compression or pressure to the center of the medial or lateral calcaneus is contraindicated during pregnancy until after the due date. Unfortunately, many practitioners and books written by non-reflexologists mistakenly misconstrue this precaution as a total contraindication to touching the heels or the feet of pregnant women. Only bone-to-bone pressure to these exact reflexes will create these negative prenatal effects.

Additionally, limit endocrine gland point stimulation to allow the hormonal orchestration of pregnancy to proceed undisturbed. Be cautious in using reflexology with substance abusers and others whose lifestyles or general health may predispose them to higher stored toxin levels, as these are believed to be released into general circulation with zone therapy.

While acupuncturists offer varying opinions on their potency, avoid similar deep, pointed pressure to the acupuncture points traditionally needled to promote uterine contractions. These include Spleen 6 (four client-finger widths prox-

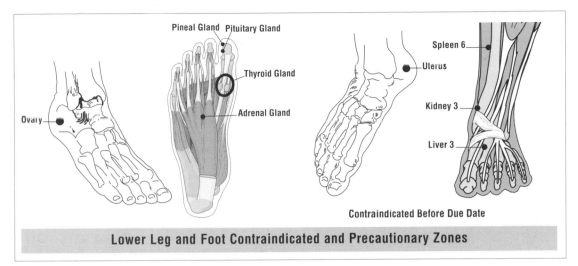

Lower Leg and Foot Contraindicated and Precautionary Zones

imal to the malleolus, along the medial tibial border), Kidney 3 (on superior border and just posterior to medial malleolus), Liver 3 (at proximal border of first and second metatarsal bones), and the complementary Hoku hand point (at the junction of the thumb and index finger). If precautions concerning clots are observed, these leg points will never be activated prenatally. Though generally regarded as less potent, address the areas of Urinary Bladder 31-34 (at each sacral sulcus) and Gall Bladder 21 (halfway between the nape of the neck and the acromium at the trapezius apex) with broad, general pressures.[42]

Passive and active movements

Women suffering nausea will not appreciate any rhythmic, rocking movements that can exacerbate morning sickness. Once nausea has passed, perform all passive movements with small amplitude, and slow, rhythmic frequency to avoid overstretching of joint structures softened by relaxin. All of a pregnant woman's ligaments are easily overstretched due to relaxin's effects. Overstretched ligaments result in joint instability and more prenatal pain. Minimally invested with elastic fibers, ligaments do not tighten after excessive stretching. Modify assisted-resisted stretches, positional release, Swedish gymnastic movements, range of motion, and other passive and active movements to prevent overstretching of joint structures. Also avoid movements that increase intrauterine pressure.

Symphysis pubis separation demands several special considerations in choosing and performing massage therapy. First, since rolling over is painful

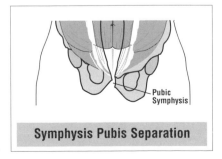

Symphysis Pubis Separation

with this condition, minimize position changes. Second, firm, reliable bolsters and other supports are essential in all positions to prevent extended tugging on the joint. Finally, eliminate any techniques that create traction on the pelvic and hip joints or that compress the pelvis unilaterally if she has symphysis pubis pain.

Other methodological precautions

When using spa treatments or other modalities involving heat, modify duration and extent of applications. Prolonged heat exposure over large body areas can increase maternal core temperatures. In the first 20 weeks, this can interfere with fetal development or even cause fetal death.[43] Saunas, steam cabinets, hot tubs, hot wraps, and other heat immersion treatments are generally contraindicated prenatally. Limit hot packs, heat lamps, and other heat modalities to local applications of less than 20 minutes. If a pregnant client becomes uncomfortably hot, or if her oral temperature rises one degree or more (Fahrenheit), discontinue heat treatment. No modifications in use of cold are required pre- or perinatally. Both hot and cold applications are appropriate during labor. (See Chapter 4.)

As previously advised, study with a master practitioner and/or instructor prior to working with expectant women. Consult with the client's maternity healthcare provider to coordinate appropriate care and secure needed releases. Take a thorough, general health history, and always observe pertinent, general contraindications for any somatic method used with a pregnant client. Follow any restrictions issued by a client's prenatal healthcare provider. Never diagnose, provide treatments for illnesses, or otherwise exceed scope of practice. Provide referrals for medical and psychological treatment. Other specific massage contraindications follow in the sections on high-risk factors and complications in pregnancy.

General Summary of Methodological Precautions and Contraindications by Trimester

Methodology	Trimester	Precaution/Contraindications
Abdominal Massage — any method	I	• Eliminate in first trimester as liability precaution.
	II & III	• Superficial effleurage and gentle rocking only.
	I - III	• Liability precaution with hypertensive disorders, premature labor, miscarriage, or placental dysfunction symptoms or risks.

Methodology	Trimester	Precaution/Contraindications

Swedish Massage	I III	• Precautions for varicose veins:
		  Mild (visible/ropy) and/or spider veins: use only appropriate Swedish and lymphatic drainage strokes at moderate pressure.
		  Moderate (palpable/raised, ropy): use only appropriate Swedish and lymphatic drainage strokes using a light touch.
		  Severe (palpable/raised, purplish/bruised surrounding tissue): use only featherlight touch; use procedures that help relieve pelvic congestion.
		• Precautions for clots (thrombi):
		  • Direct strokes toward heart.
		  • Drain proximal areas first.
		  • Use soft, whole-hand pressure.
		  • Avoid deep, pointed, or ischemic pressure into the medial border of the tibia, the saphenous area of the knee, and along or posterior to the sartorius muscle.
		  • Avoid percussion (tapotement) on legs.

	III	• All Swedish and lymphatic techniques contraindicated with underlying heart conditions.
Leg Massage	I - III	• See precautions above for legs. • Also avoid acupressure, cross-fiber friction, deep tissue, trigger points, or other deep pressure, especially to medial leg. • Contraindicated for clients on bed rest and those with increased clot risks.
Reflexive Therapies	I - III	• Reflexology: Contraindicated to uterus and ovaries; precaution to endocrine gland points; caution with substance abusers. • Acupressure: Avoid Spleen 6, Kidney 3, Liver 3, and Hoku; caution on sacrum and apex of shoulder.
Deep Tissue	I - III	• Avoid in abdomen; use only on structures chronically stressed by pregnancy; observe precautions for varicose veins and clots as above in Swedish; avoid in cases of unregulated dibetes.
Passive & Active Movements	I II & III I - III	• Rocking movements contraindicated with nausea. • Rocking movements contraindicated with nausea; caution on hips and legs with symphysis pubis separation. • Avoid hyperextension of joints.

The diagram for Swedish Massage labels: Iliac vein, Femoral vein, Saphenous vein.

Consult master teachers of somatic practices prior to applying techniques pre- and perinatally. Observe any restrictions issued by prenatal healthcare provider.

PREGNANCY COMPLICATIONS

*P*regnancy induces extensive but normal systemic changes and typical discomforts; however, some 20% to 25% of women experience unusual conditions resulting in prenatal complications.[44] These physiological imbalances can develop into complex deviations from expected physiological adaptations to pregnancy. Prenatal complications include the following: miscarriage (spontaneous abortion), ectopic or tubal pregnancy, placental abnormalities, premature labor or rupture of membranes, intrauterine growth retardation, hypertensive disorders (pregnancy induced hypertension, gestational edema proteinurea hypertension complex [GEPH], and toxemia of pregnancy), and gestational diabetes.

Your understanding of these complications and your ability to recognize their danger signs are essential. Take comprehensive medical histories and thoroughly update yourself each time you work with a woman. Be especially thorough in evaluating a woman who has a higher risk of developing these complications.

Refer women with suspected complications to their prenatal healthcare provider for diagnosis and appropriate care. Consult directly with them to determine how your work might best complement medical treatment. Partial or total bed rest is often prescribed, and massage therapy is effective in countering many of the uncomfortable side effects of restricted activity. As detailed throughout this chapter, some techniques must be modified or eliminated entirely with prenatal complications. In order to reduce legal liabilities and plan appropriate care, the prudent practitioner will secure a written medical release before proceeding with any sessions if a woman has or has had any of the complications discussed below.

Complications involving bleeding

*V*aginal bleeding, from light staining to profuse hemorrhage, can occur at any time during pregnancy, has many possible causes, and one usual maternal response — fear. Supervised massage practitioners can offer calming, comforting touch until bleeding and its cause are resolved.

In early pregnancy, bleeding sometimes occurs when the fertilized egg first attaches to the uterine wall (implantation bleeding). Within several days this bleeding will stop with no negative impact to the embryo. Vaginal or cervical sores, lesions, polyps, and anal hemorrhoids also occasionally bleed, with no direct implications for the pregnancy. A severe bladder infection creating bloody urine, however, should be treated immediately.

Bleeding related to miscarriage is, of course, serious. It may begin as staining, progressing to bright or dark red bleeding, and finally the passage of blood clots and tissue. Pelvic and/or abdominal pain and cramping are common. Appropriate medical treatment can often avert threatened miscarriages, while those termed "inevitable" have progressed beyond intervention. Most spontaneous abortions expel the entire uterine contents. Occasionally the fetus dies in utero and may not be expelled for many weeks or may require surgical removal when its death is discovered.

Miscarriage is most common in the first trimester primarily due to chromosomal abnormalities; however, spontaneous abortion may occur at any gestational age. (See previous abdominal massage section for other causes.)[45]

Both physical and emotional trauma increase the possibility of miscarriage and other complications. While motor vehicle accidents account for the majority of trauma-engendered pregnancy losses, falls, burns, and wounds from weapons are also common causes. Estimates of the frequency of battering in pregnancy range from 8% to 25% of pregnancies, and this is often an unrecognized or unreported cause of miscarriage.[46] Domestic violence stemming from increased stress levels, jealousy, and power dynamics provoke abdominal injuries and sexual abuse, and may lead to improper medical and nutritional care of the pregnant woman. Battered women are more prone to substance abuse, depression, and suicide attempts.[47] General emotional stress is also associated with higher miscarriage rates.[48]

Other causes of early bleeding include trophoblastic diseases and ectopic pregnancy. In trophoblastic diseases, placental cells develop and sometimes overdevelop despite a blighted embryo. These pregnancies are not viable, nor are ectopic pregnancies where the embryo implants outside of the uterus, usually in a fallopian tube.

Premature separation of the placenta from the uterine wall (placental abruption) threatens the life of both mother and baby. It usually occurs after the twentieth week, most often in the third trimester. As part or all of the placenta detaches from its implantation site, maternal vessels lose their placental connections and begin to bleed. Abruptions range in severity from undetectable and partial, non-endangering mild tears, to moderate separations that usually threaten the baby. In a smaller percentage of severe abruptions, massive bleeding creates fetal loss, maternal shock, and possibly death. Placental separations most commonly develop in women with chronic or pregnancy-induced hypertension, and in women who have had more than five babies. Abdominal traumas, cigarette smoking, cocaine use, and all teratogenic exposure also cause abruptions, as do uterine and umbilical cord anomalies.[49]

An even rarer placental abnormality characterized by painless bleeding, especially in the third trimester, is placenta previa. Instead of normal implantation in the upper dome of the uterus, the placenta lies near or over the cervix. Women most likely to experience previa are those carrying multiples, or are hypertensive, diabetic, or addicted to drugs, including nicotine. Endometrial damage from a prior previa, abortion, cesarean birth, or many, closely-spaced pregnancies also cause low implantation. Placenta previas often migrate by term, resulting in a higher likelihood of a normal labor and birth; if not, then a cesarean section is performed.[50]

Regardless of the cause, women experiencing bleeding often require special emotional and physical support from their massage practitioner. Stress reduction while awaiting test results and/or while on restricted activity until bleeding has resolved is especially appreciated. When pregnancy loss results, these women need not only regular postpartum care, but also assistance in their grieving process. (See postpartum care, Chapter 5.)

Vaginal bleeding in weeks 21-36 may also be a danger sign of premature labor; it is usually accompanied by symptoms of abdominal and/or pelvic pain and cramping due to regular uterine contractions continuing over an hour and with sufficient power to dilate the cervix. Early preterm labor often begins with a dull pain in the lower back that may be rhythmic or constant. As discussed previously, carefully question any client complaining of lower back pain about other possible symptoms, including pelvic pressure or a full feeling in the pelvis or posterior thighs and any change in vaginal discharge. In distinguishing between soft-tissue pain and pain from uterine contractions, remember that a positional change will usually relieve musculoskeletal pain, whereas, if labor has begun, changing position or activity usually will have no effect.[51] With written release, massage the woman with threatened preterm labor to reduce her stress, nurture her, and increase her comfort level with bed rest or other medical procedures necessary to delay labor and protect the baby.

Complications involving ruptured membranes

Vaginal discharges are normally more profuse and somewhat viscous during pregnancy. In 10% of pregnancies, however, the bag of waters (amniotic sac) ruptures before the onset of labor. A gradual trickle or a sudden gush of clearer fluids indicates that the membranes surrounding the baby have broken. Premature rupture often occurs in women who have suffered physical trauma or who have excessive amniotic fluid. If a woman suspects that her waters have broken, she needs immediate evaluation: ruptured membranes increase the risk of premature labor, infection, and umbilical cord compression.

Intrauterine growth retardation and reduced fetal movement

*T*hree percent to 10% of American babies are tinier than they should be for the length of time they have been developing. Small for gestational age syndrome (SGA) or intrauterine growth retardation (IUGR) is most common in poorly nourished mothers, drug users, and poorly controlled insulin-dependent diabetics. These babies are at higher risk for premature birth.[52]

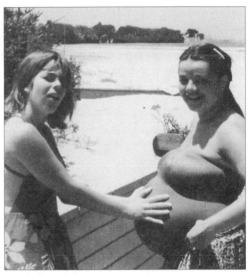

While their growth may remain normal, other babies indicate distress by reduced intrauterine movement. Most women can definitively identify fetal movement by 22-24 weeks, and they delight in their baby's familiar patterns of activity. Many women note that intrauterine movement typically stops during a fetus's 20-40 minute sleep cycles and gradually increases at night. Women who note a change in their baby's intrauterine activity patterns, especially decreased movement, need evaluation by their maternity healthcare provider.[53]

Hypertensive disorders of pregnancy

*H*igh blood pressure in pregnancy or pregnancy-induced hypertension (PIH), can degenerate to gestational edema proteinurea hypertension complex (GEPH or preeclampsia) and eclampsia (toxemia) when left untreated. While the hypertensive disorders are among the most common complications in pregnancy, experienced by 25% of American women, eclampsia is much more rare. Eclampsia is among the most serious prenatal complications, leading to permanent damage or death of both mother and fetus.[54] Those most likely to develop PIH are women of low socioeconomic status; first-time mothers (primagravidas or nulliparous); teens and those over 35; women of African descent; diabetics; and those with Rh incompatibility, and kidney and heart diseases. Women whose mothers had preeclampsia or whose earlier pregnancies were complicated by hypertension also are more likely to develop some degree of hypertensive disorder.[55]

While the causes and the process of hypertensive disorders are still unclear, the symptoms are easily recognizable. In addition to elevated blood pressure readings, women report rapid weight gain of retained water evidenced by swelling in the face, hands, and feet. Lab tests indicate spilling of protein in her urine. As the disorder worsens, edema becomes systemic and pitting, and the kidneys and liver malfunction. At its most severe, eclampsia of pregnancy involves neurological symptoms such as violent headaches and vomiting, visual disturbances of spots and flashing light, and convulsions.

High blood pressure decreases placental blood flow mandating increased practitioner caution to position these clients for maximum fetal circulation, i.e. left sidelying position. Another symptom of eclampsia, of particular note for massage therapy practitioners, is the occurrence of persistent, severe mid-back pain, especially on the right side and extending into the right shoulder, or pain mimicking heartburn. These discomforts are referred from the malfunctioning liver and, like most organically-induced pain, are not usually relieved by a change in position or activity. Carefully interview all women with this type of pain to discover any other warning signs of GEPH. Refer women with symptoms of hypertensive disorders to their maternity healthcare provider. Women with more severe symptoms need immediate medical care to prevent permanent organ damage, premature labor, fetal damage or loss, or death.

Gestational Diabetes

*D*iabetes precipitated by the physiological stresses of pregnancy is a metabolic disorder affecting approximately 5% of pregnancies.[56] It most often develops in the second trimester and is characterized by excessive hunger and thirst, frequent urination, and sugar in the urine detected in lab tests.

Pregnancy tends to increase the need for glucose in order to ensure a constant supply to the fetus. Both estrogen and progesterone stimulate increased pancreatic insulin secretion to transport glucose to the cells. In the second and third trimesters, the pregnancy hormones, human placental lactogen and cortisol, also assist in regulating blood sugar. These increased demands and the actions and interactions of these hormones can result in either the inability of the pancreas to produce sufficient insulin or the inefficient use of available insulin. Gestational diabetes is different from several classifications of diabetic conditions that may develop in childhood, adolescence, or adulthood, and which are unrelated to pregnancy. (See high-risk pregnancies.)

Those at most risk for developing gestational diabetes have a family history of diabetes and an obstetrical history of babies over nine pounds or previous stillbirths. They tend to be over 25 years old, obese, hypertensive, and have a history of skin, genital, or urinary tract infections. Those carrying twins or triplets are also more prone to developing diabetes. Gestational diabetes increases the likelihood of excessive amniotic fluid and can lead to additional complications, including GEPH, premature membrane rupture, and stillbirth.[57]

> *"I was initially alarmed when I developed gestational diabetes, but my therapist helped calm me. She taught me to breathe more deeply, and I was better able to tune into my body signals. That helped me to better notice blood sugar fluctuations and to eat according to my nutritionist's guidelines."* — Andrea

Prenatal Complications Summary

Condition	Common Symptoms (one or several may occur)	Practice Implications*
Miscarriage Ectopic pregnancy Premature labor Premature membrane rupture	vaginal discharge bleeding low back and/or pelvic pain cramping/contractions pelvic or thigh pressure	
Placental abnormalities	bleeding cramping/contraction	left sidelying position only increased clot precautions for legs
IUGR/SGA	low weight gain decreased fetal movements	left sidelying position only
PIH Disorders (hypertension, preeclampsia, eclampsia, toxemia)	high blood pressure protein in urine rapid weight gain systemic edema violent headaches severe vomiting visual disturbances mid-back pain, especially right side convulsions	* All prenatal complications necessitate the following protocols: • Comprehensive history and progress records • Written medical release • Referrals for diagnosis and treatment • Communications with physician/midwife • Modifications when on extended bed rest • No abdominal massage
Gestational diabetes	excessive hunger and thirst frequent urination sugar in urine	

HIGH-RISK PREGNANCIES

*W*omen with high-risk pregnancies are some of the most gratifying and appreciative clients to work with. Massage therapy can greatly facilitate stress reduction, ease the discomforts of frequently prescribed bed rest, and may improve the pregnancy outcome.

Physicians consider a pregnancy to be high risk when there is a greater than average likelihood of increased complications, injury (morbidity), or death (mortality) for the mother, the baby, or both. Fortunately, the usual incidence of prenatal complications is generally low; therefore, even a woman at higher risk is still quite likely to have a normal pregnancy and a normal baby. Although less than 20% of women are in high-risk categories[58], take a thorough medical history on every pregnant client. Few maternal or fetal risk factors can be impacted positively or negatively by massage protocols and techniques; however, interact conservatively with these pregnancies, and modify your sessions appropriately. Coordinate care and communicate with prenatal health care providers. Secure a written medical release with all high-risk clients to maximize effective care and to minimize legal liabilities.

Factors Considered High Risk In Pregnancy

Mother's age under 20 and over 35 (some sources specify under 17 and over 40)

Complications in previous pregnancies

Three or more consecutive spontaneous abortions (miscarriages)

Multiple gestation

Maternal illnesses: diabetes mellitus; chronic hypertension; cardiac, renal, connective tissue, or liver disorders

Rh-negative mother, or genetic problems, including DES (diethylstilbestrol) exposure, and other uterine abnormalities

Fetal genetic disorders

Drug or other hazardous materials exposure[59, 60]

Maternal age

*A*lthough most teens are physically strong, many have poor nutrition. Because smoking, alcohol, and other drug use is more common, their babies are often small, premature, and more likely to have genetic problems. Teen pregnancies are more prone to GEPH. Often their labors are also complicated, and they have higher infant and maternal mortality rates than other age groups.[61] Sixty percent of teenage mothers have been sexually abused, and the associated emotional and physical trauma often leads to further complications.[62]

While most women over 35 can expect to have a healthy, normal pregnancy, older mothers may have more underlying health issues that contribute to similar complications as teens.[63] Also, because their ova are older, genetic abnormalities are more common for mothers over 35, and therefore miscarriage rates are higher.[64]

Previous pregnancy problems

*I*f a woman has had complications in a previous pregnancy, chances are higher that she will have similar or additional problems with subsequent pregnancies. Repeat miscarriages are common, especially if she's already suffered more than one.[65]

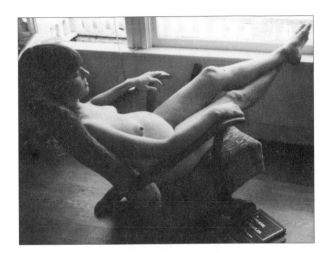

Multiple gestations

*T*win and triplet gestations significantly increase the risks of many complications, including PIH dysfunctions, gestational diabetes, placenta previa, malpresentations, small for gestational age, premature labor, and perinatal and fetal complications.[66]

> *"Because I was carrying triplets, I was on total bed rest from week 22 until their birth at 35 weeks. I got so stir-crazy and was either in pain or generally achy all the time. The last weeks I got by with my massages — they were the highlight of each week. I never would have carried my babies as long without it; massage helped me maintain the pregnancies, and my sanity."* — Beth

Maternal illnesses

*P*regnancy generates additional physiological stresses on women with chronic conditions such as diabetes mellitus, hypertension, or other pulmonary, cardiac, liver, connective tissue, or renal disorders. Increased physiological demands exacerbate many of these conditions and create additional strain to compromised organs.

Since 1920 when insulin became available, fetal mortality for diabetics decreased from nearly 98% to 5%, about the same as non-diabetics. Maternal survival rates similarly improved. This is, of course, provided that glucose is controlled both before and during the pregnancy by diet, exercise, and/or insulin injections.[67]

Despite this remarkable improvement, diabetics are still twice as likely to develop PIH and GEPH, especially if renal and vascular problems already exist; placental abruptions are often the result. Severe metabolic disturbances occur if the diabetic mother vomits excessively. Ten percent of pregnant diabetics develop excess amniotic fluid (polyhydramnios) that can prematurely rupture membranes, and increase the risk of infection. All organ systems are more susceptible to infection, especially the urinary system. Premature labor and miscarriage are more common, and the diabetic is more likely to have a cesarean birth.[68] Possible deleterious effects on fetal growth and development include congenital defects, large for gestational age (macrosomia), delayed lung maturity, hypoglycemia, learning disabilities, childhood obesity, and diabetes.[69]

Preexisting chronic hypertension increases the likelihood of placental abruption and insufficiency, as well as GEPH. With the increased load on the heart, increased blood volume, and hormonal effects, other forms of cardiac disease contribute to life-threatening complications during pregnancy. Some of the more common heart conditions requiring close medical management include rheumatic fever, valve and heart deformities, and dysrhythmias. Women with these conditions are more likely to develop thrombi, aneurysms, and heart failure. There are several classes of cardiac disease risk groups, and their mortality rates range from 1% to 50%.[70] Fetal risks are equally grave, including miscarriage, prematurity, growth retardation, central nervous system damage, and perinatal death.[71]

It is in the last trimester that blood and interstitial fluid volumes create the greatest strain on the heart. Women with cardiac disease or malfunctions are usually on bed rest, or must restrict activity from week 28 to term. Note that massage therapy techniques that increase cardiac workload are contraindicated at that time, especially Swedish and lymphatic drainage methods.

Common symptoms of chronic kidney disorders (generalized edema, proteinurea, hypertension, and decreased urinary volume) usually worsen when prenatal eclampsia develops. For the small percentage of women with this disorder, total renal failure is likely. Other diseases that significantly impact kidney function, including diabetes, hypertension, and systemic lupus, usually require close observation and evaluation during pregnancy. Severe renal disease can lead to intrauterine growth retardation, central nervous system damage, or fetal death.[72]

Women prone to kidney and bladder infections are ten times more likely to have prenatal urinary tract infections than those without such a history. Infection compromises the vital filtering functions of the kidney and can predispose the woman to preterm labor.[73] Because urinary tract infections (UTI) can also permanently damage the kidneys, encourage clients with UTIs to seek early, aggressive treatment. Avoid therapy positions and techniques that increase intrauterine pressure. Women with liver disorders, such as hepatitis and cirrhosis, are at greatest risk when GEPH or eclampsia further compromise liver function.

Several autoimmune-mediated disorders of connective tissue have serious consequences for pregnancy. The most dangerous collagen vascular disorders are disseminated or systemic lupus erythematosus (SLE), rheumatoid arthritis, and scleroderma. SLE creates an inflammation of connective tissue, most problematic in the renal, cardiac, and central nervous systems. Pregnancy outcome for both mother and baby are most severely compromised if the disease is not in remission at conception. Spontaneous abortion, worsening of symptoms, placental malformation and insufficiency, preeclampsia, thromboembolism, or preterm labor are common in as many as 60% of SLE patients. The postpartum period is risky as well.[74] Rheumatoid arthritis can precipitate cerebral and cardiac thrombi, and women with scleroderma are at higher risk of hypertension.[75]

Other maternal conditions

*A*s with most of these high-risk categories, practitioners working with pregnancies involving Rh incompatibility should be aware of the fetal risks involved. Blood hemolytic incompatibility between the mother and fetus is often fatal to the fetus when untreated. Fortunately, modern screening and treatment with RhoGAM® (rhesus gamma globulin) has decreased the risk of fetal anemia, jaundice, cerebral palsy, mental retardation, or death due to attack of the fetal blood cells by the mother's antibodies.[76] No modifications to therapy protocols are necessary with these clients, although a medical release is still recommended.

Uterine abnormalities, including an incompetent cervix, predispose a woman to miscarriage and/or preterm labor. Women born during the 1940s and 1950s whose mothers took diethylstilbestrol (DES) to prevent miscarriage suffered a high incidence of cervical malformations due to exposure to this drug. An incompetent cervix due to surgery, disease, injury, or excess relaxin, and a double uterus (septate uterus) create similar risks.[77] Observe all precautions and contraindications detailed earlier for preterm labor and miscarriage.

Hereditary fetal disorders/Drug and hazardous materials exposure

*W*hile massage therapy has no effect on genetic disorders, practitioners should note that these pregnancies are at higher risk for miscarriage and premature labor.[78] These pregnancies include hereditary disorders, such as sickle-cell anemia and Down's syndrome, and conditions caused by viral, drug, or environmental factors that cause fetal malformation. Consumption of alcohol, cocaine, or nicotine, or exposure of mother or father to other hazardous substances also increases the risk of fetal deformities, miscarriage, prematurity, and low birth weight.[79]

Other cautionary conditions

*C*ertain health problems, while not considered high risk by the American College of Obstetricians and Gynecologists, predispose women to pre- and perinatal complications. Observe caution when clients are without prenatal care, or have asthma, anemia, or convulsive disorders. A lifestyle involving smoking, drinking, drug use, poor nutrition, or multiple sexual partners often fosters a problematic pregnancy that is more prone to complications.

As many as 27% to 55% of American women have survived childhood sexual abuse. During pregnancy and labor, these women may reexperience aspects of their earlier trauma such as genital injury or pain, fear, anger, shame, defensiveness, loss of control, isolation, disassociation, or repressed memories.[80] They may require additional emotional support, and often benefit greatly from respectful and nurturing professional touch. Various professionals believe that sexual abuse as a child or teen doubles the risk of prematurity and neonatal complications.[81]

When other conditions generally considered contraindications to massage therapy occur prenatally, modify sessions accordingly.

CONCLUSION

*S*ome sobering facts of American maternity care are very relevant to somatic practitioners: more than 75% of obstetricians and gynecologists are sued; more than 33% of them are sued more than three times; and nurses and other perinatal healthcare providers are more and more frequently being included in these lawsuits.[82] Somatic practitioners are wise to be aware of the litigious atmosphere in childbearing and to conduct responsible, ethical practices.

More importantly, no practitioner wants to have any doubt as to whether their work was harmful or their protocols questionable. This may best be ensured by following all safety recommendations of this text and of clients' healthcare providers; by practicing conservatively and conscientiously within the scope of somatic therapies; and by pursuing a comprehensive pre- and perinatal massage therapy education. Practitioners can then expect to effectively and safely facilitate the development and health of both baby and mother.

Chapter

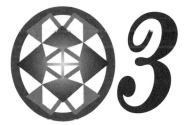

3

Trimester
Recommendations

*E*very woman's pregnancy is a unique experience that follows predictable developmental stages. Each three month trimester is typified by common changes shared by many pregnant women. These adaptations are exquisitely programmed to foster a healthy pregnancy, and often they result in challenges to a woman's physical and emotional resiliency. To respond appropriately to both her individualized and characteristic needs, somatic practitioners must understand and respect these changes. Each trimester requires specific considerations for positioning and safety protocols.

With modifications, virtually all therapeutic massage and body-work methods are applicable prenatally. In this chapter, a variety of effective therapeutic somatic activities are suggested. Pursue qualified instruction in these methods prior to using them during the childbearing year. In addition, sidebars detail the most essential techniques for nurturing the births of mothers and their babies. The author's comprehensive certification workshop further develops these and 75 other specific pre- and perinatal massage techniques (See Resources appendix).

FIRST TRIMESTER (WEEKS 1-13)

Watching the pregnancy test stick indicate "positive," a woman confirms what her tender, swollen breasts and her queasy stomach have been intimating to her for the two weeks since her menstrual period was due. She's pregnant!

An intricate sequence of hormonal communications has already begun preparing her body for the nine months of creative activity ahead. Human chorionic gonadatrophin (hCG), detected in home urine tests, ensures adequate first trimester hormonal levels. Though diminished after week 14, hCG continues to protect the fetus from rejection as foreign tissue.[1]

The hypothalamus, pituitary, thyroid, parathyroid, adrenal glands, and ovaries enlarge, and accelerate hormonal production that creates extensive physiological adaptations. Estrogen, progesterone, and other pregnancy-specific hormones are also manufactured by the placenta. They stimulate positive changes that increase fuel, and vitamin and mineral supplies, ensuring sufficient maternal energy levels and robust fetal growth. These changes include increased energy storage in the form of fat in the thighs, buttocks, and abdomen. Progesterone relaxes smooth muscle linings of (1) the digestive tract, thus maximizing intestinal absorption time and uptake of iron, calcium, and other nutrients; (2) the uterine muscles, to prevent excessive, premature contractions; and (3) the vascular walls, to maintain a healthy, low blood pressure.[2]

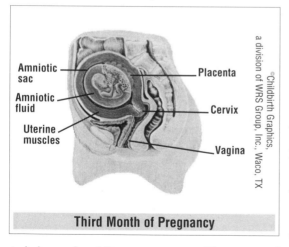

Amniotic sac
Amniotic fluid
Uterine muscles
Placenta
Cervix
Vagina

©Childbirth Graphics, a division of WRS Group, Inc., Waco, TX

Third Month of Pregnancy

Another of progesterone's effects is increased respiratory efficiency characterized by greater tidal volume in the lungs and faster respiratory rate to handle increased cardiac output. Meanwhile, estrogen stimulates uterine growth and blood supply; balanced salt, water, and insulin levels; and increased metabolic efficiency in sugar and carbohydrate utilization.[3]

These vital hormonal adaptations are evidence of the body's wisdom in sustaining a healthy pregnancy. They are also responsible, in part, for an initial three months of exhaustion, urinary frequency, and, often, morning sickness.

In this first critical trimester, the embryo grows from a microscopic fertilized egg into a three-inch fetus weighing one ounce. It has a developing body, eyes, ears, and a beating heart. As the fetus grows, so does the supportive placenta, usually firmly implanted on the upper, posterior uterine wall. Infused with estrogen, the uterus itself grows to one-third larger than normal, from plum to grapefruit size. Its upper edge (fundus) is palpable half way up to the umbilicus by 13 weeks.

Though her abdomen may not look identifiably pregnant in this first trimester, the pregnant woman's waistline thickens. Her sensitive breasts continue to swell, and pressure on them is often painful. In these early weeks, the expectant woman may feel unusually tired. After one or two naps each day, she may collapse early in the evening for nine or ten hours sleep; however, frequent urination brought on by hormonal influences will probably interrupt this much-needed sleep.

First Trimester Maternal Concerns

Enlarged, tender breasts

Emotional and hormonal adjustments

Fatigue

Frequent urination

Morning sickness or all day nausea and/or vomiting

Some women experience no nausea. Fifty percent to 88% have a very queasy stomach in the morning or early evening, and many are hypersensitive to smells.[4] She may even suffer nausea and vomiting all day during this time. While unpleasant for the mother, one evolutionary biologist, Margie Profet, has theorized from her work with plant toxins that this may offer some evolutionary benefit. Morning sickness may prevent women from ingesting toxins that cause fetal malformations in this developmentally critical first trimester. She suggests that women follow their instincts toward blander foods to ease morning sickness.[5]

Structural stresses to her body are minimal in these first 13 weeks, except to the cervical and thoracic spine and to the pectoral girdle. Increased breast size initiates an inexorable anterior shift in her center of gravity. Toward the end of this first trimester, the thoracic spine and rib cage may begin to collapse with the weight of the breasts, and the pectoral girdle may tend to rotate anteriorly, further compressing the rib cage. Her head shifts forward with the chin more raised. As her body makes these postural adjustments, a woman whose pre-pregnant posture is swaybacked may begin tilting her pelvis even farther forward, hollowing her lower back.

While the first trimester woman is usually overjoyed, even the most desired pregnancy may prompt fear, worry, regret, or sometimes anger or a fatalistic feeling. She is embarking on a transformative journey that will leave no part of herself unchanged. Fear of miscarriage or debate about abortion may distract her, as well as guilt about drug use, lifestyle choices, or health issues.

Pregnant women commonly experience fluctuating emotions (lability) including: doubt, fear, loneliness, anger, apprehension, changes in sexual response, or disgust with her body. She may feel trapped, exposed, inadequate, more dependent or independent, joy, triumph, excitement, and/or fulfillment. Typical worries about the actual birth that may begin to percolate include: pain; fear of failure, injury to the baby, loss of control and autonomy or loss of dignity; fear of hospitals, insufficient or poor medical care; inadequate spousal support; or genital mutilation.

Other emotional issues childbearing women may need to explore involve "last egg in the basket," sexual or spousal abuse, stirred memories of life issues and traumas, abortion, miscarriage, prematurity, deformity, cesarean birth, "wrong" sex, death, high-risk factors, infant illness, single parenting, and/or worries about older children.

Their partners often are happy and anticipatory but may also feel isolated, trapped, jealous, angry, disconnected, fearful, and worried about failure, financial stresses, rejection, older children, and/or stirred memories of life issues and traumas.[6]

♦ ♦ ACTIVE LISTENING ♦ ♦

A supportive, nonjudgmental environment created by the sensitive practitioner provides opportunities for women to openly and honestly express the full range of emotions engendered during pregnancy. Emotional support is especially critical for those who are alone in their pregnancy, due to the emotional or physical absence of their partners. Follow these guidelines to actively listen, to encourage her self-understanding, and to offer emotional nurturing.

1. Establish rapport with direct, calm eye contact, empathetic words, and receptive body language that conveys interest and concern.
2. Be alert to what is being said, how it is being said, and what is left unsaid to fully and accurately understand the client.
3. Acknowledge what she shares; clarify and summarize for accuracy and to increase her self-understanding.
4. Invite more exploration by appropriate, open-ended statements, such as "How did you feel then?", "Where do you experience that feeling?", "Tell me more about that."

5. Identify any incongruent information, expressions, body language, or feelings. Be alert to the "charged" content, words, and phrases that feel "hot", "tender", "tense", or "soft."

6. Do not offer unsolicited advice, and limit your own storytelling, unless requested to share.

—————— ♦ ♦ ♦ ♦ ——————

Considerations for practitioners

Only minor adaptations in positioning on the therapy table are necessary in the first trimester. To increase comfort in the prone position, use cushions with breast recesses. Some women's breasts will be too tender for her to lie face down, even with such additional support. Remember to use pillow or bolster support under the knees to reduce lumbar curvature when in supine position.

In the early weeks of pregnancy, focus massage therapy on relief for fatigue, nausea, and other physiological adjustments. Expect the newly pregnant woman's need for relaxation and empathetic listening to be high. Many women eagerly request self-care information, reading recommendations, and guidance in preparing for the months ahead. (See appendix for recommended reading list.) Encourage her to consult with her healthcare provider, and begin appropriate exercises for pelvic floor and abdominal strengthening[7, 8, 9] and for stretching of tight muscles.

Schedule massage sessions at the time of day when the pregnant woman is most comfortable and least nauseated. Use only unscented oils, or fragrances that she finds appealing. Aromatherapists recommend six drops of lavender essential oil to four ounces of massage oil as stimulative to cell growth, a sedative for insomnia, and for relief from headaches, cystitis, and yeast infections. It is also reported to both strengthen contractions and reduce labor pain, particularly when in combination with clary sage, ylang ylang, and rose.[10] Suggest that she empty her bladder immediately prior to her session.

Remember to observe all contraindications and precautions detailed in Chapter Two, especially:

♦ No abdominal touching (legal precaution).

♦ Avoid reflexive pressure to points stimulating the uterus when working on the legs, feet, hands, sacrum, and upper back.

♦ Avoid rhythmic rocking movements when she's nauseated.

♦ Limit techniques on the medial leg to soft, whole-hand pressure.

♦ Use a gentle, yet firm touch with all techniques moderated to an experience of pleasure on the borderline of pain as maximum depth.

Prenatal complication symptoms are a contraindication to working with a pregnant woman until she provides a written release from her physician or midwife. Be particularly alert to the possibility of miscarriage, ectopic pregnancy, and GEPH, particularly for first-time mothers (primagravidas). Observe other contraindications generally relevant for massage therapy.

Safe Positioning for First Trimester Massage Therapy
Supine
Prone
Sidelying
Semireclining
Seated

♦ ♦ SOMATOEMOTIONAL INTEGRATION ♦ ♦

While most women discuss feelings within the normal conversation of a therapy session, sometimes stronger emotional expression occurs. Because intense emotional processing releases stress hormones into both maternal and fetal circulation, this type of cathartic release is best limited to integral issues that naturally surface and will potentially detract from the pregnancy and birth if left unresolved.

When working with clients who are experiencing strong feelings, remember the following:

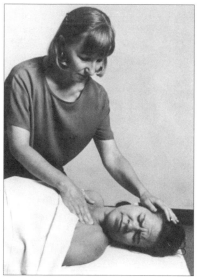

1. Maintain both your own and your client's breathing. Calm, center, and relax with diaphragmatic breathing. Accelerated breathing, breath holding, shallow, and paradoxical breathing all increase emotional agitation.

2. Support your client's ability to uncover her feelings with receptive, not overly directive, guidance.

3. Use subtle contact, deep pressure, or gentle, rhythmic rocking to facilitate emotions surfacing. Clients typically restrict expression at the solar plexus; anterior-lateral neck; chin and jaw; immediately lateral to the nose; the eyebrows; immediately

inferior to the clavicles; and the medial thighs and feet.

4. If she becomes distressed, help her to remain present and grounded with contact that focuses on her physical sensations. Work on her legs and feet, guide her to slower, deeper breathing, and repeat and validate her insights.

5. Stay alert and flexible in response to her needs. Provide safety, reassurance, environmental comforts, safe positioning on the table, and movement options.

6. Allow time for assimilation and reorientation to normal reality.

7. Encourage emotional support through family, friends, self-help groups, clergy, or psychological professionals. Remember to follow up with her yourself.

8. Many psychological dynamics are outside of the massage therapist's or bodyworker's scope of practice and expertise. Establish a reliable network of professionals who are knowledgeable and experienced in working with childbearing women.

♦ ♦ ♦ ♦

♦ ♦ ACUPRESSURE FOR MORNING SICKNESS ♦ ♦

Teach clients to stimulate the Pericardium 6 (PC-6) acupuncture point to decrease nausea and morning sickness.

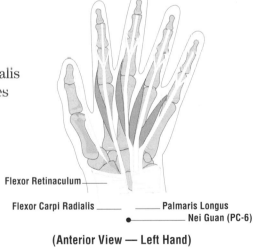

1. Locate the PC-6 point between the most lateral two tendons on the anterior surface of the forearm (flexor carpi radialis and palmaris longus tendons), two inches proximal to the wrist crease.

2. Apply deep, rhythmic thumb or fingertip pressure to these points on each arm four times daily for ten minutes each application.[11]

Flexor Retinaculum

Flexor Carpi Radialis _____   _____ Palmaris Longus
                               _____ Nei Guan (PC-6)

(Anterior View — Left Hand)

♦ ♦ ♦ ♦

Summary of recommended first trimester bodywork

Women in their first trimester will benefit most from the following therapeutic somatic activities:

♦ **Body-use education** in diaphragmatic breathing, pelvic positioning, iliopsoas development, and other postural alignment and structural balancing; appropriate abdominal strengthening activities; strengthening and awareness of the pelvic floor musculature, especially by Kegel exercises.

♦ **Experiences of deep relaxation, internal focus, and awareness**, through touch, visualizations, and other relaxation techniques.

♦ **Cross-fiber friction, deep tissue, lomi-lomi, passive movements, trigger point, and stretching techniques** to reduce strain to the joints and soft tissue of the upper spine and pectoral girdle, especially the scapulo-thoracic and rib cage joints and the following muscles: trapezius, rhomboidei, erector spinae, levator scapulae, supraspinatus, and pectoralis major and minor.

♦ **Nurturing, gentle touch** to reduce stress and to create a supportive, caring experience.

♦ **Nonjudgmental, active listening** to assist her in processing feelings and emotional issues that she may be experiencing. Provide appropriate referrals to other professionals as needed.

♦ **Swedish, lymphatic drainage, craniosacral therapy, zone therapy, acupressure, and/or other reflexive techniques** to assist in circulation, reduce stress and fatigue, relieve nausea and other digestive disturbances, and facilitate general physiological processes.

"My work with Allison actually began in the 18 months prior to her first successful pregnancy. She had just miscarried after 10 years of trying to get pregnant, including extensive fertility treatments. How sad and angry she was! A 'caretaker' and hard worker, she wanted to clear her feelings, become more in tune with herself and her true goals, and more receptive to her natural fertility. Over the course of our bi-monthly sessions, with committed lifestyle changes, and after a session when she yielded to her image of her nurturing grandmother, she conceived again. We evolved, together, a visualization of her breath encircling this baby protectively inside her. We focused on relaxation, particularly in her legs, pelvis, and computer-cramped neck and upper back. What an achievement and joy for her to deliver her naturally conceived daughter later that year!" — Carole Osborne-Sheets, integrative body therapist, San Diego, CA

"Katherine's initial experience in her first pregnancy was typical: nausea, fatigue, and generalized anxiety. Some days she could minimize the morning sickness with careful eating and by working the acupressure point I showed her. She asked many questions about pregnancy and self-care, and she consumed every recommended book. While working on her tense neck and upper

back, she cried briefly — excited, happy tears mixed with fearful sobs. What would happen to her and her marriage, she wondered.

Because she had had juvenile arthritis, as well as a mild scoliosis, we worked in these first sessions on maximizing her postural integrity to minimize joint strain later in the pregnancy. It wasn't until the second trimester, however, that she felt well enough to begin stretching and strengthening her back and abdominals." — Sandy Jackson, neuromuscular therapist, San Diego, CA

SECOND TRIMESTER (WEEKS 14-26)

While tiredness, nausea, and other physical and emotional changes characterize the first trimester, the pregnant woman usually enjoys weeks 14 through 26. Many women feel as though their pregnancies, especially these three months, are the most vibrant and vital times of their lives. By this point she has adjusted hormonally and has adapted her nutrition, exercise, and daily routines to nurture her pregnancy. She has an identifiably pregnant contour. Her baby's rhythmic heartbeat and subtle, first movements confirm the reality of her pregnancy.

She may, however, begin to feel additional structural stresses as her posture adjusts to increased weight and a shift in her center of gravity. Her baby will grow in this trimester to between 11 and 14 inches, weighing about one and one half pounds. Increased to melon size, her uterus reaches her umbilicus. With this growth, her abdominal and lumbar musculature may become fatigued.

Chronic shortening begins to develop in the posterior myofascial sheath, or superficial back line. This articulated myofascial chain, that extends from the plantar surface of the foot, along the paravertebral musculature, to the skull, is one of the main "anatomy trains" described by Rolfer, Thomas Myers.[12] As normal balance among the abdominal, iliopsoas, and paravertebral muscles diminishes, maintaining good posture is more difficult, and she may experience some pelvic and back pain. Muscles and ligaments around the hip joints also begin to strain as the femur sustains more lateral rotation in the acetabulum. She also may feel compressed in these joints, and in her knees and feet, depending on the amount of weight she has gained.

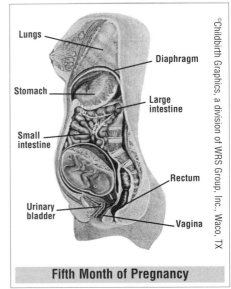

Lungs

Diaphragm

Stomach

Large intestine

Small intestine

Rectum

Urinary bladder

Vagina

©Childbirth Graphics, a division of WRS Group, Inc., Waco, TX

Fifth Month of Pregnancy

The uterus not only grows in the second trimester, but it also floats higher out of the pelvic cavity and more into the abdominal cavity. This change usually allows more room for the urinary bladder to fill, bringing some relief from the first trimester's frequent urination. Unfortunately, this growth also may produce intermittent, sharp pain in her lower abdomen, groin, and perhaps down one leg as the uterine round ligament stretches. Referred pain in the lumbar and gluteal musculature from the uterine broad ligaments is also common. She also may begin to hyperventilate and suffer heartburn in this trimester.

As her uterus and breasts grow, the second trimester woman may discover that her skin feels taut, itchy, and becomes, perhaps, stretched to the point that prominent lines appear on her abdomen, breasts, buttocks, or thighs where the connective tissue and the skin have torn. These stretchmarks (strae gravidarium) will fade somewhat after the pregnancy.

She also may notice many other estrogen-related effects. Some women have increased skin oiliness, acne, and/or hair loss or texture changes, while most enjoy smooth, clear, radiant skin and hair. A thin brown line from the pubic bone up to the umbilicus (linea negra) will darken on her now protruding abdomen. Her areola, nipples, and vulva will become even bluish black, depending on her skin pigmentation. A "mask of pregnancy" (cloasma) with dark splotches over her forehead, nose, and cheeks may appear. She may develop spider veins and/or varicose veins, depending on the extent of increased blood volume, her activities, and hereditary predisposition.

Second Trimester Maternal Concerns
Pregnancy seems more real
Increased weight
Back, pelvic, hip, and leg pain may develop
Round and broad ligament pain
Stretchmarks
Skin and hair changes
Varicose and/or spider veins
Constipation and/or heartburn

Varicose veins in the rectum (hemorrhoids) may cause her some discomfort as well. Not only does progesterone slow down intestinal peristaltic movements, but iron supplements, high protein consumption, decreased abdominal space for the intestines, and increased water absorption in the colon may result in constipation, strained bowel movements, and hemorrhoids.

Often the emotional highlight of the second trimester is feeling first movements and hearing the baby's heartbeat. By weeks 20-26, barely perceptible butterfly-like fluttering in her abdomen will have gradually developed into distinctive rolling, prodding, sliding, and rhythmic movements. Her baby repositions, stretches, hiccups, sucks its thumb, and otherwise plays and grows in its watery, uterine environment. With the aid of a specialized stethoscope, her healthcare provider will help her hear the brisk, strong heartbeat of her baby.

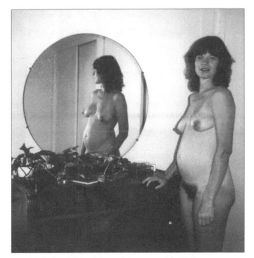

Joyous greetings and ongoing communications between the woman and her baby, and between the baby and other family members and friends, will make the pregnancy both more real and personal. But this reality may also generate financial concerns, health worries, and changes in roles and relationships with spouse, family, and friends.

Some women delight in the full, rounded appearance of their breasts, hips, and belly during pregnancy. Many women discover a new sensitivity to their bodies and relish their heightened sexual responsiveness, more typical in this trimester. The need for more comfortable lovemaking positions and, perhaps, alternatives to intercourse often opens sensual and sexual exploration.

Others may feel unattractive, even deformed. Negativity about physical appearance may surface at this time. The media image of femininity, with flat stomach, small hips, and high breasts, is pervasive in American culture. Embarrassment and negativity are likely if a woman shares this image as being her ideal. She may also endure rejection by her husband or partner as her body rounds during pregnancy.

Positioning considerations for practitioners

Adjustments for increased uterine size is a primary concern for the somatic practitioner working with second trimester women. Sacrouterine ligament strain is likely when prone, even when supported by pillows or the Contoured bodyCushion® (see Resources appendix), but especially on tables designed with a hole or separation for the pregnant abdomen. The additional weight and pressure applied to the back during prone procedures may significantly increase intrauterine pressure. (See positioning concerns, Chapter 2.) Also, encouraging relaxation in the position least favorable to structural integrity is of questionable value. As in the first trimester, increased breast size or sinus congestion also may make the prone position uncomfortable.

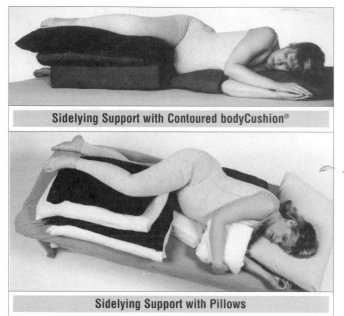

Sidelying Support with Contoured bodyCushion®

Sidelying Support with Pillows

The sidelying position is the best position for massaging a pregnant woman's back and pelvis. With the client positioned securely on her side, the practitioner may then safely apply the deep pressure that may be necessary for relieving strain and tension in the posterior structures with little fear of increasing intrauterine pressure. Use several sizes of firm and soft pillows, a long body pillow, and/or a Contoured bodyCushion® to create a foundation for a secure sidelying position. Support the woman's head so that her cervical spine is aligned with her torso, and not hyperextended or sidebent. These supports also should accommodate the space between the acromioclavicular joint and the head so that her shoulder is not uncomfortably compressed beneath her upper torso weight.

When only using pillows, tuck a small foam wedge (see Resources appendix) or pillow, approximately eight inches square and two to four inches thick, under her abdomen near the pubic bone to support the uterus and prevent uterine ligament and lumbar strain. Place another similarly-sized pillow under her waist to support the lumbar spine if her hip and waist proportions are markedly different. Provide an additional pillow in front of the chest to support her upper arm, relieving pressure on tender breasts and preventing anterior rotation of her upper body.

Extend the bottom leg, and position it on the table posterior to the other leg to avoid restriction of venous flow. For the uppermost leg, place supports of sufficient height and density to maintain a horizontal line between hip, knee, and ankle, and to moderately flex this hip and knee. This will prevent strain on the sacroiliac joints and the lumbar spine, and anterior rolling of her torso. Proper leg height also mechanically assists in the reduction of leg edema, and provides relief from painful varicose veins.

The almost fetal sidelying position offers psychological comfort for most pregnant women. Nestled comfortably on her side, she may feel more able to talk about her excitement and her concerns without the obstruction of a face cradle, as when prone, or the confrontational effect of talking face-to-face, as when supine. With the woman on her side, the practitioner may still unobtrusively observe her expressions and breathing for emotional responses.

For supine support, use an 8-10 inch wedge or pillow, two to four inches thick under the client's right side. Elevate her right side from rib cage to hip with the wedge tucked from her spine out laterally to her right side. This pillow will shift the weight of the uterus and baby off the inferior vena cava preventing supine hypotensive syndrome.[13] Place a pillow or bolster for support under her knees and head, if desired.

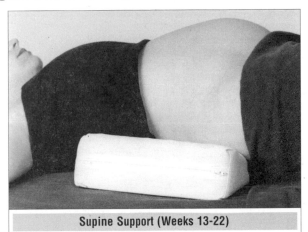

Supine Support (Weeks 13-22)

After the twenty-second week, use only sidelying, semireclining, or seated positions. In the semireclining position, she will straighten her legs with pillow or bolster support under her knees. She may then recline her entire torso against a firm foundation placed at the head end of the table. Maintain an angle (torso to table) of between 45° and 75° from her hip joint to her head. With this support, uterine weight will not compress the vena cava as it would in the supine position.

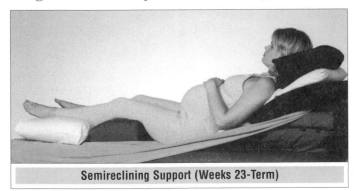

Semireclining Support (Weeks 23-Term)

Achieve semireclining support with a firm foam wedge foundation (see Resources appendix) at least 24 inches high and further padded by other pillows. Use a backjack constructed of a metal framework and canvas sling, usually used for floor sitting, or a folded Contoured body-Cushion® instead of the foam wedge. Several therapy table manufacturers also offer table models with a split top that may be elevated to several heights for semireclining positions (see Resources appendix). Use additional bolsters or small pillows to provide both the lumbar spine and the cervical spine with essential support. For added comfort and circulation, use a pillow under the calves. Most on-site massage chairs afford comfortable, safe semireclining support when the pregnant client leans back against the chest padding.

> ### Safe Positioning for Second Trimester Massage Therapy
>
> Supine, with pillow under right hip, up to 22 weeks.
>
> After 22 weeks, no supine; use semireclining, sidelying, and seated positions.

Practitioners' body mechanics

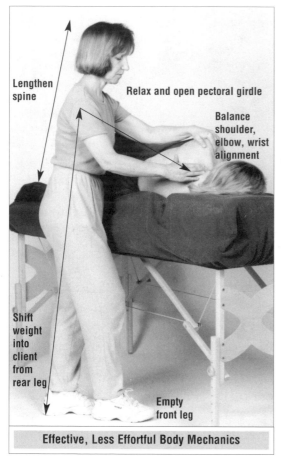

Lengthen spine

Relax and open pectoral girdle

Balance shoulder, elbow, wrist alignment

Shift weight into client from rear leg

Empty front leg

Effective, Less Effortful Body Mechanics

*A*djust table height for sidelying position so that the top is between wrist and knuckle level when standing erect at table side. Many practitioners find this to be considerably higher than when working primarily with prone or supine clients; however, this height will be more comfortable and effective for sidelying work since weight must be shifted more horizontally than downward into the table.

Begin strokes with your entire torso facing the direction of planned force and from a stable, relaxed stance. Space feet shoulders' width apart, with one foot 10 to 15 inches behind the other. Settle your entire body weight into your rear foot and leg with ankle, knee, and hip gently flexed. Apply your body weight to create pressure and depth by shifting from your rear leg into the client's body, without adding weight to your front leg. Your center of gravity will then be somewhere between you and your client as you lean into her. With these dynamics, you should be able to lift your front leg from the floor **without** any weight adjustments. Complete strokes by shifting your weight out of the client, returning all of your weight into your rear leg. By generating all techniques with your legs and directing their force with pelvic movements, your hands become the relaxed endpoint for your total body energy. Alternately, assume a "horse riding" stance parallel to the table, then shift weight between both feet, particularly when performing kneading strokes.

Lengthen your entire spine both downward and upward to maintain less stressful vertical alignment, regardless of the angle of lean or depth of pressure required. Engage the serratus anterior to maintain horizontal balance of your pectoral girdle and to prevent shoulder and neck strain. Further protect shoulder, elbow, wrist, and hand joints by neutral, balanced alignment, and by creating force from the lower body weight shift rather than pressing only with the upper body.

"The energy is rooted in the feet, developed in the legs, directed by the waist, and expressed through the fingers." — Tai Chi Classics

Practitioner guidelines and precautions

Structural stresses on the weight-bearing joints and the myofascial structures of the back and hips intensify during the second trimester. Begin and complete each session with guidance in structural balance using visualizations and kinesthetic cues. Emphasize bodywork that is effective for relieving tension and muscle strain, fibrosis, myofascial pain, muscle cramping, and joint dysfunction in the spine, and in the pelvic and pectoral girdles. Aston-Patterning® is an educational system that is particularly effective with prenatal structural stresses. Aston-Patterning® includes bodywork, movement coaching, ergonomics, and fitness training to facilitate optimal expression and function. By customizing sessions to the individual woman's interests and unique history, she learns to neutralize the effects of the past to allow new possibilities for adjusting to her pregnancy. (See Resources appendix.)

♦ ♦ PREGNANCY STRUCTURAL REBALANCING ♦ ♦

Vertical alignment of the head, spine, and pelvis reduces many of the musculoskeletal and physiological discomforts of pregnancy. Encourage balanced, effortless alignment with the following exercises.

Occipital lift

1. Verbally guide the standing client to imagine a string attached to the crown of her head and extending skyward.
2. Instruct her to imagine that the string is pulled further skyward, lifting the crown of her head with it and allowing the cervical spine, rib cage, and pelvis to follow.

Pelvic and lumbar alignment

1. Ask the client to imagine a long monkey tail attached to her tailbone and pulled between her legs, with the end at chest level where she can grasp it.
2. Verbally guide her to imagine pulling her tail to stretch it over her head, then releasing it back to the beginning position at chest height. Ask her to imagine this movement two more times, coordinating the imagined movements with her breath; inhaling, the tail is in front of her chest, and exhaling she pulls it over her head.
3. Instruct her now to continue imagining pulling her monkey tail, allowing the resulting movement of her pelvis. Encourage her to coordinate the imagery and her pelvis tilting with her breathing as above. Also guide inhibition of the extrinsic muscles and isolated use of the iliopsoas.
4. Continue gently tilting and releasing the pelvis for up to one to two minutes.
5. Encourage her to repeat pelvic tilting throughout her day, in lying, standing, and seated positions to help reduce pelvic congestion, strengthen the iliopsoas, and decrease lower back strain.
6. For other prenatal postural alignment guidelines, consult *Essential Exercises for the Childbearing Year*.[14]

♦ ♦ ♦ ♦

♦ ♦ HIP AND BACK SCULPTING / TRIGGER POINTS ♦ ♦

Relax chronic tension and reduce pain with deep, melting sculpting of the paravertebral and gluteal muscles and of the posterior fascia.[15] Myofascial release in these areas assists in spinal, pelvic, and hip realignment, eases strain to the sacroiliac, lumbosacral, and intervertebral joints, and often relieves sciatic pain. Deep, sustained pressure on the lateral pelvis helps to reduce uterine broad ligament referrals. Extinguishing trigger points uncovered while sculpting diminishes referred pelvic, lumbar, and hip pain.

1. With your client sidelying, compress unilaterally into an identified restricted area of the paravertebral myofascial structures. Sink to a level of tissue resistance, but create an intensity no more than pleasure on the borderline of pain.
2. Continue to the base of the sacrum, moving as the deeper tissue elongates, or performing a series of compressions for 30 seconds each.

3. Stand posterior to her pelvis, facing toward her feet, and use the proximal forearm or the fist of your arm closest to her feet. Slowly compress into the gluteus medius, beginning at its attachment on the inferior iliac crest.

4. Follow any myofascial release taking you deeper into the gluteus minimus or along the gluteus medius fibers. Continue performing a series of compressions for 30 seconds each until reaching the insertion in the iliotibial tract, with any movement on the skin occurring due to elongation of tissue beneath.

5. Reposition your forearm or fist to slowly compress into the gluteus maximus, beginning at its attachments on the sacrum and posterior iliac spine. Follow any myofascial release that takes you deeper or along the fibers. If there are no spider veins, proceed to its insertion and down the iliotibial tract.

6. Slowly compress into the channel between the ischial tuberosities and the greater trochanter to relax the bellies of the deep lateral rotators. Avoid pressure on the sciatic nerve which is indicated by a burning, numbing sensation in the client's posterior leg.

7. Continue by carefully sculpting their attachments around the greater trochanter.

8. As you sculpt in these areas, be alert to any points eliciting a jump response from the client or referred pain (myofascial trigger point). Check for trigger points in longisimus thoracis (T-8-10 and L-1), iliocostalis lumborum, multifidus (S-1), quadratus lumborum, gluteals, piriformis, and tensor fascia lata.

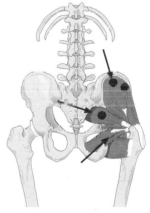

9. Moderate your pressure on an identified trigger point until the pain is no more intense than pleasure on the borderline of pain.

10. Request client feedback of changes in pain intensity. Once her pain dissipates, continue to compress for 7-20 seconds. If possible, stretch the trigger area for 30-60 seconds, or perform localized strokes over the area.

11. As an alternative to sustained pressure, move client to a position that eliminates the pain, and hold her there for 90 seconds. Slowly return her to her original position.

◆ ◆ ◆ ◆

After the first trimester, light abdominal effleurage and rocking are both soothing and safe, unless specifically contraindicated by the woman's healthcare provider, or if the risk of miscarriage or premature birth is high. Lubricants containing vitamin E oil and cocoa butter are helpful in relieving itchy, stretched skin. When combined with olive oil, elastin, collagen, and hyaluronic acid, these creams may be effective in minimizing stretchmarks.[16] Beginning in months three or four, the woman may massage and friction these products into her abdomen, hips, and thighs with a cloth twice daily to activate skin circulation.

Observe strict contraindications to massage therapy techniques requiring deep pressure into the abdomen. Strain to the abdominal and iliopsoas muscles and sluggishness in the colon are common; however, Swedish massage, deep tissue massage, neuromuscular techniques, or other techniques requiring abdominal pressure are not safe. Massage the abdomen only with light effleurage strokes that do not penetrate below the superficial fascial level. Other modalities, such as pelvic tilting, abdominal strengthening, and reflexive techniques applied on the feet or hands may promote safe relief in these areas.

Because blood clots may develop in the second trimester, avoid all techniques detailed in Chapter Two that can potentially dislodge clots and cause embolisms. Avoid these techniques particularly on the medial surface of the leg, to the femoral triangle, into the bowl of the pelvis, and just medial to the anterior superior iliac spine (ASIS). The closer to the pelvic bowl a clot forms, the more serious the consequences, so special caution should be exercised in the femoral triangle and in the inguinal region.

Avoid routine use of deep work especially on the legs. Be particularly careful to moderate pressure in areas of spider veins or varicose veins and the medial surface of the legs.

It is safest to assume that all pregnant women have asymptomatic blood clots and that, if varicose veins are visible, there may be similarly weakened, deeper veins. Gentle effleurage and kneading are appropriate on mild and moderate varicose veins. Only featherlight pressure to create lymphatic movement at the skin surface is safe on severe varicose veins that are bulging, discolored, or have lesions. Carefully apply techniques at the hips and pelvic area that assist blood flow from the legs and reduce pelvic blood and lymph congestion. Encourage her to frequently elevate her legs when sitting or lying to alleviate pooling of blood and lymph, and ease the pain from varicose veins.

Fatigue contributes to another common pregnancy discomfort, muscle cramps in the calves. Both the gastrocnemius-soleus complex and/or the peroneals may spasm, especially during the night, causing many women to awake in great pain. Passive stretches of these muscles during cramping are effective and may help to prevent spasms when used daily. The pregnant woman and her partner should learn effective stretches for the calf muscles. Also teach partners to gently effleurage her legs and feet daily. Assisted-resisted exercise, kneading, and lymphatic drainage techniques also assist in removal of waste products produced by cramping, and reduce the likelihood of recurrence. Remember to avoid compressing deeply into the medial surface of the calf during kneading. Maintain her foot in a neutral or dorsiflexed position when massaging her feet to prevent inducing a cramp.

♦ ♦ ASSISTED-RESISTED STRETCHES FOR CALF CRAMP RELIEF ♦ ♦

Perform and/or teach clients these stretches to both prevent and alleviate cramps in the gastrocnemius, soleus, and peroneals.

1. Hold the client's foot in dorsiflexion (toes toward patella) and have her gently attempt to plantar flex her foot (point her toes) while you resist this action for five seconds. Release and repeat twice, increasing the dorsiflexion slightly with each repetition.
2. Perform these movements with her knee flexed, and repeat three times with it extended.
3. Hold the client's foot in inversion (lateral edge toward her sole) and have her attempt to evert (lift the lateral edge toward her knee) while you resist this action for five seconds. Release and repeat twice, increasing the inversion slightly with each repetition.
4. When teaching her to perform stretches for herself, have her hold the ends of a towel stretched under the ball of her foot. For the peroneals, instruct her to cross one calf over her thigh so that she may hold her foot.

♦ ♦ ♦ ♦

Zone therapy on the feet can help to alleviate many common complaints: constipation, heartburn, headaches, hemorrhoids, and musculoskeletal pains. If a woman has never experienced reflexology, or is a substance abuser, exercise good judgment in using these techniques with her to avoid overwhelming her system with release of stored toxins. Remember to avoid bone-to-bone reflexive pressure at precautionary points detailed in Chapter Two. Most women thoroughly appreciate Swedish and passive movement techniques that ease aching, tired feet.

Various types of passive movements can be problematic in the second trimester. If nausea persists, continue to eliminate rhythmic passive movements from sessions. Some second trimester women will occasionally experience symphysis pubis separation. Avoid traction and large amplitude movements involving the hip joints that may exacerbate this pain.

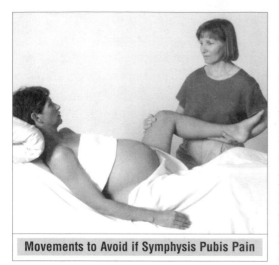

Movements to Avoid if Symphysis Pubis Pain

As in the first trimester, be alert to signs and symptoms of developing complications of pregnancy. While 85% of miscarriages occur in the first 13 weeks,[17] later miscarriages and non-viable early births can happen in the second trimester. First time mothers are more likely to develop hypertension or preeclampsia, perhaps as early as the twentieth week.[18, 19] Increased urination in the second trimester, when less frequent urination is the norm, can indicate gestational diabetes. Note symptoms of other complications and refer these clients to their healthcare providers. (See pregnancy complications, Chapter 2.)

Bed rest in pregnancy

Often women with complications or who are in high-risk categories are placed on bed rest. This can mean either total inactivity or reduced mobility with long rest periods each day. Several days or weeks or many months of these restrictions may be prescribed, depending on the woman's condition. Most of these women are confined to home while others require hospitalization.

In addition to the increased fear generated by this heightened level of concern, many women feel shocked, resentful, guilty, lonely, dependent, bored, and anxious about finances, work, and other responsibilities. Often, however, protective determination and a fierce devotion to nurturing her baby are also stimulated. With inactivity comes sluggish circulation, increased risk of thrombi, constipation, heartburn, edema, muscle strain, cramping, and stiffness.[20] Bones lose calcium, and appetite wanes.

After receiving release from her prenatal healthcare provider, visit bed resting clients in their homes or in the hospital. Most women will be able to move to your therapy table, or adjust the hospital bed to a comfortable working height. Prevent back strain when leaning over the bed by having her as close to you as is safe. Many conditions requiring bed rest, especially those involving high blood pressure and fetal circulation concerns, respond well to various massage therapy methods. Remember to support her in a sidelying position on her left side for maximum fetal circulation.

♦ ♦ DIAPHRAGMATIC BREATHING REEDUCATION ♦ ♦

Full, easy diaphragmatic breathing facilitates relaxation and increases kinesthetic awareness. Diaphragmatic breathing involves the easy, controlled use of
the anterior, posterior, and lateral sections of the diaphragm. Use the following
visualizations to guide clients toward more complete activation of the diaphragm
and maximum lateral and posterior excursion of the rib cage. If a woman
breathes paradoxically, retrain her to maximize maternal and fetal oxygenation
and to prepare for the breathing demands of labor.

1. Ask the client to place one hand on her lower abdomen and the other on the
   center of her chest.
2. Instruct her to inhale through her nose and exhale through her mouth gently
   and deeply without strain.
3. Ask her to visualize the following
   sequence in her mind's eye:
   a. See your baby nestled in your
      uterus, deep within your pelvis.
   b. Imagine that your inhaling breath
      gently touches her/him like a soft,
      loving hand.
   c. As you exhale, see the caressing
      hand of your breath gently lift
      from her/him
   d. Watch this movement as you
      continue to breathe fully for
      several minutes.

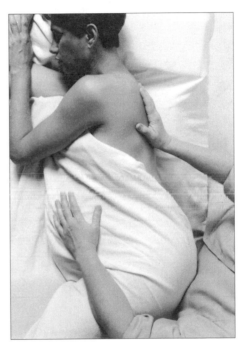

4. Observe any straining, especially any
   over inflating of the chest or activation of the scalenes and other neck
   muscles with the inhalations. Verbally
   encourage her to breathe effortlessly,
   without force.
5. Enhance her awareness by placing your hands on her torso at the specific
   areas toward which you are guiding her breath. When a client has difficulty
   visualizing, switch instead to asking her to place her hands on her abdomen.
   Ask her to lift her hands away from her spine with her inhalation and allow
   them to sink toward her spine with her exhalation, as suggested by
   Elizabeth Noble.[21]
6. Encourage frequent, daily diaphragmatic breathing and relaxation.

♦ ♦ ♦ ♦

Improve circulation of women on bed rest with Swedish and lymphatic drainage work; however, eliminate leg strokes due to increased risk of clots. Reduce musculoskeletal pain with appropriate myofascial, passive movement, stretching, and trigger point techniques. Calm, center, and nurture her with focused, gentle touch, reflexology, selected craniosacral or other relaxing techniques. Many women especially enjoy foot, head, and neck massages for relaxation.

With approval of her doctor/midwife, encourage her to gently stretch and exercise in bed. Raising her hips off of the bed in a bridging movement, curl-ups, leg sliding, and ankle circles help to maintain conditioning and improve sluggish circulation.[22] Assisted-resisted stretches both relax and help maintain strength in the involved muscles. Emphasize stretches of the arms and legs. Encourage her to seek guidance in the use of light weights to improve muscle tone.[23]

Allow generous time for sharing of feelings and companionship needs. Celebrate each day's or week's progress toward her goal of a healthy baby. Listen empathetically when she expresses her frustrations and fears. Journal writing is particularly soothing and integrating for some women.[24] Encourage her to use this "time out" to tune in to her baby, to have her physical and emotional needs fully met, and to meditate or pray. Teach her family and friends simple massage techniques, providing thorough safety guidelines.[25] Suggest books, videos, and other educational media, and help her focus on her inner journey to motherhood with selected books, such as *Cradle and All: Women Writers on Pregnancy and Birth*[26] and *The Book of Birth Poetry*.[27] Offer to connect her with support groups specifically organized to assist pregnant women on bed rest such as Sidelines National Support Network. (See Resources appendix.)

Whether or not on bed rest, any pregnant woman who experiences a symptom of a complication should obtain a written medical release from her prenatal care provider before massage therapy. Additionally, observe general contraindications to massage therapy.

Exercise during pregnancy

*A*ppropriate exercise fosters healthy mothers and babies. Well-designed prenatal exercise maintains strong postural musculature, prepares specific muscles, and develops endurance for the exertions of birthing.[28] It may even contribute to decreased labor pain by boosting production of natural pain relieving hormones (endorphins).[29] Aerobic conditioning optimizes a woman's fitness level and general health. Because of scope of practice limitations, practitioners should encourage their clients to seek consistent exercise in accordance with the recommendations of their physician or midwife. Be prepared with suggestions of books, videos, and local, qualified prenatal exercise instructors.[30-34] Design your somatic sessions to encourage clients' postural integrity, labor preparation, and kinesthetic awareness.

The American College of Obstetricians and Gynecologists (ACOG) advises expectant women not to exceed a heart rate of 140 heartbeats per minute, or 70% of maximum heart rate, whichever is less, while exercising for a maximum of 15-20 minutes. Safe limits may be 140-160 beats per minute in well-conditioned women. Target heart rate is measured by this calculation: (220-Age) x .70 = target heart rate. Pregnant women can safely exercise for more than 20 minutes at a time, but not at an aerobic level.[35]

According to Elizabeth Noble, prenatal physical therapist and exercise instructor, a maximum of 45 minutes of mild to moderate exercise, including a warm-up and cool-down period, will usually prevent maternal core temperature from exceeding 100.4°F or 38°C. Because excessive heat taxes the fetus' limited thermoregulatory capacity, extended, vigorous exercise may cause neural tube defects. Continuous, rhythmic, large muscle exercise also can lead to shunting of oxygen away from fetal circulation possibly causing fetal oxygen deprivation. Safe aerobic exercises, particularly for previously sedentary women, include stationary cycling, walking, and swimming. Competitive and dangerous sports are not recommended.[36]

The hormone relaxin affects all of the ligaments, tendons, and muscles prenatally, creating ligamentous laxity. Pregnant women should avoid deep knee bends, overextension of the neck, elbows, wrists, lower back, hips, and knees, and overstretching in any position. Lifting light weights (1-3 kg, 2-5 lb) promotes muscle toning while preventing injuries to joints and ligaments. Additionally, to avoid any potential risks, she should not vigorously exercise in the supine position, especially longer than five minutes; hold her breath or strain during exercise; perform jerky (ballistic) movements; or stand motionless for prolonged periods.[37]

Summary of recommended second trimester bodywork

*P*regnant women in weeks 14-26 will derive the most benefit from the following therapeutic somatic activities:

♦ **Body-use education** in diaphragmatic breathing, pelvic tilting, iliopsoas development, and other postural alignment and body usage instruction; appropriate abdominal strengthening activities; strengthening and awareness of the pelvic floor musculature, especially by Kegel exercises.

- ◆ **Experiences of deep relaxation, internal focus, and awareness**, through touch, visualizations, and other relaxation techniques.
- ◆ **Cross-fiber friction, deep tissue, lomi-lomi, positional release, structural balancing, passive movements, trigger point, stretching, and connective tissue massage techniques** to reduce strain to the joints and soft tissue of the upper and lumbar spine, especially the sacroiliac, lumbosacral, scapulo-thoracic, rib cage, and hip joints, the superficial back fascial line, and the erector spinae, intrinsic spinal extensors and rotators, hip rotators, trapezius, rhomboidei, levator scapulae, supraspinatus, pectoralis major and minor muscles.
- ◆ **Myofascial and postural alignment activities** to relieve pain from strain to the round, broad, and sacrouterine ligaments of the uterus that stretch greatly in this trimester.
- ◆ **Nonjudgmental, active listening** to assist her in processing feelings and emotional issues she may be experiencing. Be especially alert to concerns about body image, sexual activity, her health and/or the baby's development, changes in relationships, dependence and independence, abuse, and previous problematic pregnancies. Provide appropriate referrals to other professionals as needed.
- ◆ **Nurturing, gentle, touch** to reduce stress and create a supportive, caring experience.
- ◆ **Swedish, lymphatic drainage, craniosacral, zone therapy, acupressure, and/or other reflexive techniques** to assist circulation, reduce stress and fatigue, relieve gastrointestinal discomforts, and facilitate general physiological processes.
- ◆ **Swedish, stretching, connective tissue massage, and appropriate deep tissue work** to assist in preventing and/or relieving developing varicose veins, cramps, and fluid buildup in her feet and legs.

> *"I have had the honor of working with two "multiples" moms through the entire second half of their pregnancies; one carried twins, and one triplets. In both cases we started with bi-monthly sessions, and we moved into weekly sessions by the twenty-sixth week.*
>
> *I was amazed at the incredible changes that these pregnant bodies withstood. Both moms were on strict bed rest and retained fluid in what seemed to be gallon amounts. Their backs ached as their bellies swelled to accommodate the growing babies. They got less and less sleep as their due dates approached. Their limbs trembled as they walked because of lack of exercise. They both wound up*

wearing their husbands' biggest slippers to protect their puffy feet when they left the house for their doctors' appointments.

In the last months of their pregnancies, they both told me that the only way that they could make it through the three days prior to our sessions was to live minute by minute, and to constantly remind themselves that I was coming again soon. The three days following our sessions would be more comfortable for them, and then the cycle would start again. Unfortunately, financial circumstances did not permit more visits per week. (I was already doing house calls for a fraction of my in-office fee.)

I am pleased to report that the twins made it just past 40 weeks of gestation, and the triplets up to 36 weeks. Both moms firmly believe that without massage therapy, they would have delivered much earlier. They have told me that both the physical and emotional nurturing that they received helped carry them and their babies longer than usual in multiple pregnancies. I am delighted to have had a part in nurturing these remarkable women and their babies, and I look forward to doing so again in the future."
— Liz Ellis, massage therapist, Chicago, IL

"I have one client who will always remain close to my heart. At the time of her pregnancy, she was a single mom who was sent to me by her social worker. This was an older woman who had just graduated from college with high honors, but she was feeling very depressed over her personal life, especially over the pregnancy. At that time she could not love her unborn child. As we worked together during the last six weeks of her pregnancy, I was able to sense her body beginning to relax as her endorphin levels increased with the massage. The more relaxed she became, the more she began to talk about her baby. By the time the baby was born, she was in love with it. By the way, she had a very easy, unmedicated labor. She was admitted to the hospital about two hours before she gave birth." — Carroll Patterson, massage therapist, Austin, TX

THIRD TRIMESTER (WEEKS 27-40+)

*P*regnancy's final months and weeks often are bittersweet for a woman as she longs to bask in the feeling of her newborn in her arms, yet is reluctant to move ahead to this new life phase. Her anticipation grows as she and the baby dramatically increase in size. In the third trimester, her baby's weight will more than triple to a typical seven and one half pounds by birth. Its length will almost double to 20 inches. All organ systems are developed by the eighth month, with the exception of the lungs.

This dramatic fetal growth increases anterior weight load and often results in typical musculoskeletal strain and discomfort for the mother. Sacroiliac and other lumbar joint and myofascial pain may create moderate to severe discomfort. Increased strain, not only to the round ligament, but also to the broad and sacrouterine ligaments of the uterus, may result in referred pain in the buttocks and lower back. (See detailed structural adjustments, Chapter 1.)

As the uterus enlarges, the band of fascia dividing the rectus abdominis (linea alba) conveniently separates allowing space for the rapidly maturing baby. While usually not painful in and of itself, this diastus further weakens the already stretched muscle. Without the rectus abdominis to assist in pelvic alignment, the iliopsoas is usually no longer capable of maintaining vertical pelvic orientation. The lumbar spine finally collapses into excessive curvature (lordosis).[38] Additionally, she may begin to waddle rather than activate the psoas for hip flexion when walking.

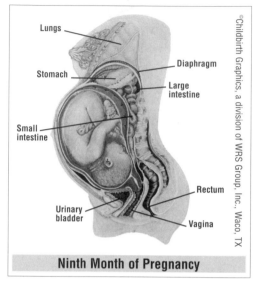

Ninth Month of Pregnancy

Increasing relaxin levels will continue to prepare her pelvis to accommodate the emerging infant. This may mean less pain for those with fibromyalgia and tight ligaments, but these last weeks of higher relaxin levels may create separation of the symphysis pubis, with resultant pain in the center of the pubic bone. Walking, rolling over on a therapy table, standing from a seated position, and getting in and out of a car will cause pain.

Third Trimester Maternal Concerns	
Eagerness and anxiety	Edema in feet and legs
Weight gain	Wrist or hand pain
Increased back, pelvic, and hip pain	Leg cramps and "restless leg" syndrome
Diastus recti	Varicose veins
Symphysis pubis separation	Urinary frequency
Hyperventilation	Braxton-Hicks contractions
Heartburn, constipation, hemorrhoids	Lightening

During this last trimester, she will likely experience some edema or fluid retention in her feet and legs, a normal response to the 40% increase in interstitial fluid volume. As the weight of the uterus increases pressure in the femoral veins, varicose veins also may occur. For some women, pain, tingling, or numbness will occur in the hand or wrist as a result of either edema-induced carpal tunnel syndrome or posturally-induced thoracic outlet syndrome.

Because the fundus will reach the rib cage, the third trimester woman will become increasingly short of breath due to decreased lung space. Her stomach and intestines are compressed as well, so heartburn, hiatal hernia, and constipation with resulting hemorrhoids are common discomforts. The later weeks of pregnancy may bring the pregnant woman some welcome relief from shortness of breath. This comes when her baby prepares for labor by dropping lower into her pelvis, its head "engaged" against the cervix. However, increased urinary frequency may also result as the baby's head compresses her urinary bladder to less than one-third its normal size.

As her due date approaches, her uterus will begin "practice contractions" (Braxton-Hicks) as the uterine muscle fibers tense irregularly for 15-30 second intervals. While these contractions are usually light, some women find them mildly painful. Changes in activity and position usually will dissipate these contractions. These "false labor pains" accomplish only minimal cervical dilation and effacement, but they do begin to prepare her psychologically for laboring.

Labor begins only if these early contractions dilate the cervix to two centimeters, last 30 seconds or longer, become more rhythmic, and continue for 4-20 minutes. Because prematurity is one of the major causes of newborn complications and deaths,[39] the baby may be at significant risk if labor occurs prior to 37 weeks of gestation. Evaluation by her maternal healthcare provider is essential if she suspects that she is in premature labor.

With labor and birth imminent, the pregnant woman may become impatient and restless, increasingly eager to be done with her pregnancy. Many women begin to "nest" by cleaning, arranging, and otherwise readying themselves for the birth. It is important that she not overtire herself at this time. Frequent "time-outs", rest, and relaxation are essential.

In her book, *Celebration of Birth*, Sheila Kitzinger, noted British social anthropologist, birth educator, and author, speaks of the experience of many third trimester women:

> *A woman with child, melon-ripe, peach-firm.*
> *Blood, grape-red, rushes in her veins*
> *swirls in the cavern of her pelvis*
> *pours through placenta and pulsing cord.*
> *She sees, hears, smells, touches more keenly*
> *with animal vitality.*
> *She is a ship sailing on a swelling sea*
> *toward a sure harbor.*[40]

On the other hand, fears for the baby's or her own health may dominate her dreams and thoughts. Thousands of women's dreams have been studied revealing unusually vivid, often bizarre yet universally meaningful prenatal dreams. Forty percent of studied women reported awakening from terrifying nightmares, and fearful elements dominated another 30% of women's dreams. Though many women hide such dreams, encourage them to discuss their fears and make preparations to minimize the likelihood of occurrence. Actively "incubating", or deliberately dreaming, guided imagery, and visualizations stimulate resolution of fears, diminish feelings of victimization, and may reduce labor time.[41]

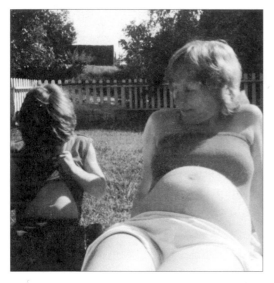

If labor seems to begin prematurely, she may feel unprepared and worried. Many women are concerned about medical interventions, whether medically necessary or imposed upon her as standard procedures. She may desire to have the birth proceed in a certain way and experience "performance anxiety." She may have to take leave from her job, or give up other responsibilities and activities earlier than anticipated, creating financial or emotional strain. Births of older children may have been traumatic so that she is anxious about this impending birth.

Pregnancy and birth are sexual experiences in the broadest sense. Physically, the sexual organs are intensely stimulated and engorged with blood. She may feel emotionally sexual and inspired with feelings of great love, joy, surrender, and giving. This implicit sexuality may be energizing for her, as expressed by many of the women in veteran midwife Ina Mae Gaskin's book, *Spiritual Midwifery*,[42] but it also can be unsettling. Physicians and other attendants touch and examine her, inserting their hands and instruments into her vagina. She must assume revealing positions, some of which she may not consider comfortable even in the privacy of her darkened bedroom.

The sexual nature of pregnancy and birth can be particularly stressful for those women who have experienced sexual abuse and trauma in their past. Victims of childhood sexual abuse, assault, and rape often cope with their experiences by abandoning physical awareness, detaching themselves physically and emotionally, and by repressing memories and feelings. The intensity of pregnancy and birth can bring these hidden feelings to the surface and create conscious or unconscious emotional stress — vague whispers or tearful torrents of sadness, anger, and fear.[43]

She also may be awash in joyous anticipation of her baby. Her dreams may be of tender images of her child at her breast and of her expanded family "in love." Preoccupied with ideas for girl's and boy's names, she may increasingly focus inward in a soft, warm reverie of creativity as she watches and feels her baby swirling within her, ever closer to its birth. Respectful sensitivity to the depth and range of all of these emotions is essential for the somatic practitioner.

Positioning considerations for practitioners

*D*uring weeks 27 to term, position pregnant women on the therapy table only in the sidelying or semireclining positions. As previously discussed, prone positioning creates too much intrauterine pressure and strains the sacrouterine ligaments. Extended supine positioning, even with a small pillow under the right torso and hip, creates too much risk of restricted blood flow to the uterus. (See second trimester positioning concerns, Chapter 3.)

Since many women labor in the semireclining position, becoming accustomed to this position and learning to achieve maximum relaxation here will help her labor preparation; however, New Zealand midwife Jean Sutton, and Pauline Scott, childbirth educator, argue convincingly from their extensive practices that regular semireclined sitting in late pregnancy encourages a higher incidence of posterior fetal presentation often resulting in long, painful labors.[44] (See prolonged labor, Chapter 4.)

Safe Positioning for Third Trimester Massage Therapy

Sidelying, semireclining, and seated only

Practitioner guidelines and precautions

*S*tructural stresses on weight-bearing joints during the third trimester usually cause a woman's most intense discomforts. Most women will welcome relief of chronic tension, myofascial pain, and muscle cramping. Erase trigger points, and utilize deep tissue, cross-fiber friction, passive movements, and other forms of therapeutic bodywork in the following areas: posterior spinal structures, rib cage, posterior pelvis (especially the lumbosacral and sacroiliac joints), hip and thigh movers, hip joints, upper torso, neck, and pectoral girdle. Limit deep tissue massage to areas that are directly stressed by the pregnancy.

With increased structural stresses, third trimester women benefit greatly from postural alignment and body-use reeducation. Encourage numerous and frequent repetitions of the pelvic tilt to strengthen the iliopsoas muscle, reduce lumbar lordosis, and decrease lower back and abdominal muscle strain. By the third trimester, compensation for increased anterior weight load has usually created a pronounced posterior lean of the upper rib cage and anterior displacement of the head on the spine. Teach her to regularly correct these two postural distortions, and she will suffer less pain in the upper back and neck, as well as increase her ability to breathe more deeply.

♦ ♦ LUMBOSACRAL STRETCH (PASSIVE PELVIC TILT) ♦ ♦

A passive pelvic tilt will stretch the lumbosacral and intervertebral lumbar joints and surrounding myofascial tissue. It will facilitate the client's ability to correctly maintain pelvic/spinal alignment and reduce hip, lumbosacral, and sacrouterine ligament strain and pain.

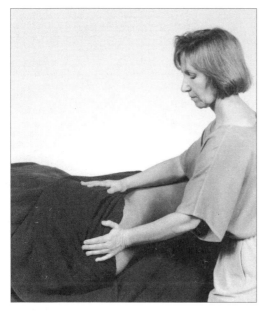

1. With the client in sidelying position, stand behind her lower back. Cover her sacrum with your fist or the palm of your hand nearest her feet. Place your other hand on her anterior superior iliac spine (ASIS).
2. Stretch the lumbosacral joint as you passively rotate the pelvis. Apply firm, anteriorly directed pressure to the sacrum that turns the coccyx, as though tucking a tail. Allow the hand on the ASIS to remain relaxed.
3. Hold this stretch for 30 seconds to one minute. Add rhythmic, small amplitude rocking of the pelvis, if desired.
4. If common tender points between the first/second, and second /third sacral spines are present, apply anterior directed pressure to the apex of the sacrum and hold for 1-2 minutes.
5. Teach her to actively reposition her pelvis. (See pregnancy structural rebalancing, second trimester section of this chapter.)

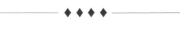

◆ ◆ SACROILIAC RELEASE ◆ ◆

The following blend of deep tissue sculpting and rhythmic passive movement creates myofascial relaxation and reduces compression and rotation of the sacroiliac (SI) joint.

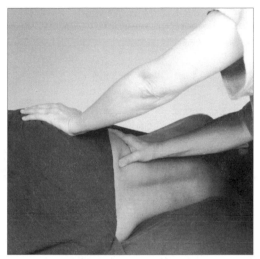

1. With the client in sidelying position, stand at lumbar level facing her feet. Use fingertips or thumb to compress toward the SI joint of the higher hip. Sink just medial to the posterior iliac spine. Compress to a level of tissue resistance, but create an intensity no more than pleasure on the borderline of pain.

2. While maintaining this pressure, place the palm of your other hand between her sacrum and greater trochanter. Initiate gentle traction toward her knee accompanied by subtle, small amplitude rocking that shifts her ilium away from the sacrum.

3. Maintain this simultaneous pressure, traction, and rocking for a minimum of 30 seconds.

◆ ◆ ◆ ◆

Many women find relief from the weight of the uterus by gently cupping their hands under their abdomen just superior to the pubic bone to hold the baby's weight with their arms. Others may choose to use supportive undergarments, a prenatal support belt (see Resources appendix), or fabric wrapped in the styles of many traditional cultures to support the abdomen and ease back pain. Supporting the uterus can also reduce venous pressure that contributes to varicose vein development in the legs. Reduce varicose vein pain by including modified Swedish leg work in each session, emphasizing raking and light vibrational techniques.[45]

One of the most common needs of the third trimester woman is relief from edema, particularly in the feet and legs. Relieving myofascial restriction in the inguinal area will increase blood and lymph return from the legs. This is accomplished by correcting her vertical alignment, by encouraging numerous pelvic tilts, and by performing limited, specific myofascial procedures. Positional relief also will be effective, both on and off the therapy table, as will lymphatic drainage and gentle, modified Swedish techniques on the legs. Acupressure to the medial arch four times daily may reduce edema in the feet.[46]

Tapotement and deep work on the legs, especially the medial surface, and in the inguinal area are increasingly dangerous in the third trimester when the risk of developing and dislodging thrombi is highest. Continue to avoid reflexive touch to labor stimulating points on the feet and hands. Remember that women with underlying heart conditions may not safely receive Swedish or lymphatic work in the last trimester.

If calf cramps occur, relieve them as in the second trimester. With increased weight gain, some women develop hip, knee, foot, and "restless leg" pain. "Restless leg" is usually felt as an irritating achiness that gradually intensifies when she is resting and usually causes an intense need to shake and/or rub the affected leg. Since both leg cramps and "restless leg" are primarily manifestations of physiological imbalances in nutrients, salt, water, and hormones, suggest consultation with a nutritionist or her healthcare provider to supplement Swedish massage therapy and stretching.

Symphysis pubis separation is more common in the third trimester. To prevent increasing pelvic pain, avoid techniques that pull on this joint. If a woman has symphysis pubis pain, eliminate position changes on the table to prevent exacerbation of her discomfort. Include positional release techniques that realign the joint. Though uncommon, if nausea occurs, avoid rocking passive movements.

If she experiences carpal tunnel symptoms, thoroughly drain the arms and hands with Swedish and lymphatic work and maximize space in the carpal tunnel with gently, small amplitude mobilizations and traction. Be alert to possible development of GEPH. Encourage her to wear a wrist splint to hold her wrist in slight flexion and to elevate it overhead on pillows while sleeping. For hand and arm pain of thoracic outlet syndrome, focus on postural realignment activities and relief of chronic tension in the scalene and pectoralis minor muscles. Craniosacral, especially thoracic inlet release, strain and counterstrain, and other passive movements to the rib cage and pectoral girdle are also effective.

Stretched skin and muscles in the abdomen will benefit from gentle, rhythmic effleurage to lubricate the skin and ease strain. Usually the baby will respond to this contact on the walls of its home with distinctive kicks and squirms. Deeper pressure into the abdomen still is contraindicated.

♦ ♦ RIB CAGE RELEASES ♦ ♦

Reduce myofascial tension and tender trigger points in the intercostals and rib cage attachments of the abdominals. Rib cage expansion is then more comfortable, and deep abdominal breathing is easier. With less myofascial restriction, postural realignment of the rib cage and spine is more effective. Extinguishing trigger points will also reduce referred back pain.

1. Stand beside your sidelying or semireclining client at waist level and facing her shoulder.
2. Using the flat of your fingertips of your inside hand, reach between her abdomen and breast to contact the distal border of the rib cage at xiphoid level.
3. Lean away from the client to gently sink into the myofascia on the rib cage. Avoid pressure into her abdomen by remaining on the distal cartilage. Do not slip inferiorly or curl your fingertips under the rib cage.
4. Wait a minimum of 30 seconds for myofascial release that allows a sculpting movement along the distal border or deeper into the tissue.
5. Continue deep tissue sculpting laterally and discontinue when you discern the floating eleventh rib.
6. Apply oil and reposition your hand to sink superficially while creating a sawing motion with your finger tips into the external obliques, the rectus rib cage attachments, and serratus anterior. "Saw" deeper into the intercostals of ribs 6 through 10.

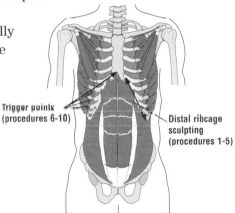

Trigger points
(procedures 6-10)

Distal ribcage
sculpting
(procedures 1-5)

7. As you make repeated passes in these tissues, seek any points eliciting a jump response from the client or posterior or anterior rib pain. These trigger points are most prevalent in areas of soft tissue dysfunction and spasm.
8. Moderate your pressure on an identified trigger point until the pain is no more intense than pleasure on the borderline of pain.
9. Request client feedback about changes in pain intensity. Once her pain dissipates, continue to compress for 7-20 seconds.
10. If possible, stretch the trigger area for 30-60 seconds, or perform localized strokes over the area.
11. Alternately, move the client to a position that eliminates the pain, and hold her there for 90 seconds. Slowly return her to her original position.

♦ ♦ ♦ ♦

In her book, *Enhancing Lamaze Techniques*,[47] Janice S. Novak recommends that third trimester pregnant woman strengthen the abdominal muscles by performing sit-backs rather than curl-ups. By the eighth and ninth months, most women will not be able to do curl-ups. Additionally, since third trimester women should not exercise on their backs for any reason, sit-backs are the recommended form of abdominal strengthening. In a sit-back, a woman sits a short distance from a wall with her legs apart, supported by pillows under the knees. As she exhales, she leans towards the wall, keeping a straight back. Maintaining tension in her abdominal muscles, she uses an eccentric contraction of the rectus abdominus muscle to "brake" against her own body weight. On the return, she uses her arms to push back to a sitting position, avoiding direct strain on the rectus abdominus.

Novak also outlines the following procedure as support for the almost inevitable separation of the rectus abdominis muscle in the third trimester. Before a sit-back is performed, the pregnant exerciser places the fingertips of both hands at the lateral edges of her rectus, on the opposite sides of her body, at about umbilical level. When the rectus is activated in the sit-back, she gently pulls medially with her fingertips to hold the two sides of the rectus together.

Be alert to any edema in areas other than her feet and legs, especially the face and hands, as warning symptoms of possible metabolic imbalances. Until the woman's physician or midwife gives written permission, no work should continue if systemic edema, or any other symptoms of GEPH, toxemia, gestational diabetes, premature labor, or placental dysfunction occur. (See complications, Chapter 2, and bed rest section, Chapter 3.)

Premature labor, or rhythmic tightening and contraction of the uterus prior to 37 weeks gestation, can result in birth of an underdeveloped infant. Since premature labor may include the common third trimester complaint of low backache, question clients concerning occurrence of other labor symptoms such as rhythmic pelvic or thigh pressure, abdominal cramping, or vaginal discharge. If pain persists, regardless of position or activity, this may be an indication of possible premature labor or kidney infection rather than musculoskeletal problems. With any combination of these indicators of premature labor, withhold massage therapy until receiving written release from the client's healthcare provider.

LABOR PREPARATION

*I*n addition to relief from common pregnancy discomforts, during weeks 32 through 40, focus therapy on labor preparation, including practicing relaxation; preparing the pelvic floor for birth; increasing flexibility in the hips and legs so that she may labor in a variety of positions; teaching diaphragmatic breathing and visualizations to facilitate labor; increasing kinesthetic awareness; offering opportunities to process feelings and increase communication skills; and improving her ability to relax through intense stimulus and pain.

Pelvic floor preparation

The muscles of the perineal area act as a supportive sling for the pelvic organs and as sphincters for the urethra, vagina, and anus. Most women do not have well-toned pelvic floors, and pregnancy further strains them as they must support the enlarging uterus and maintain bladder control.

When the baby's head descends through the vagina and "crowns," or appears at the vaginal opening, the muscles, connective tissue, and skin of the pelvic floor must stretch tremendously. Without adequate stretching, she may tear, or the birth attendant may have to surgically enlarge the vaginal opening (episiotomy). Frequent and numerous exercises of these muscles (Kegel exercises) from early pregnancy, and perineal massage beginning later in the third trimester, will prepare the pelvic floor for birth.[48] Kegel exercises also reduce the likelihood of postpartum urinary stress incontinence and promote healing of episiotomies, perineal tears, and anal and vulvar hemorrhoids.[49]

In *The Birth Partner*,[50] noted childbirth educator, Penny Simkin, P.T., describes the conditioning of the pelvic floor muscles as consisting of two components. toning and bulging. Toning is accomplished by contracting the pelvic floor as though simulating the movement necessary to stop the flow of urine, or to hold a walnut in the vagina. A pregnant woman should tighten her pelvic floor for five to ten seconds for a recom-

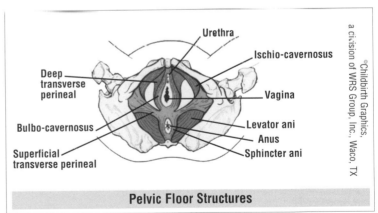

Pelvic Floor Structures

Urethra
Ischio-cavernosus
Deep transverse perineal
Vagina
Bulbo-cavernosus
Levator ani
Anus
Superficial transverse perineal
Sphincter ani

©Childbirth Graphics, a division of WRS Group, Inc., Waco, TX

mended 100 times throughout each day. She should try to breath normally and allow the leg, buttock, and abdomen muscles to remain relaxed while doing these exercises.

Letting go of these same muscles during labor will allow the baby to be born. Simkin suggests that pregnant women rehearse for crowning by consciously bulging out the pelvic floor at the end of a Kegel. This is accomplished when she holds her breath and **gently** strains as though she were having a bowel movement. Alternately, as she contracts her pelvic floor, she may imagine that it is like an ascending elevator. As she releases the contraction, the "elevator" descends gradually. She bulges the pelvic floor by imagining the elevator reaching basement level. In the last six weeks of the pregnancy, she should increase her emphasis on the bulging phase of Kegels.

Simkin and many other childbirth professionals also recommend the use of prenatal perineal massage to prepare the perineum for birth. While this form of internal vaginal massage is inappropriate for massage practitioners to perform, many women are interested in learning massage techniques that they or their partners may do to prepare the perineal area. Utilizing the webbing between thumb and index finger to replicate the perineal tissues, teach interested women to perform perineal massage on themselves in preparation for birthing. Studies have indicated that improving the conditioning of the perineum may reduce the need for episiotomy and the occurrence of lacerations. Women who do not massage their perineum are almost two and a half times more likely to tear than those who perform appropriate perineal massage.[51]

The woman or her partner should perform daily perineal massage in the last four to six weeks of the pregnancy. (If a herpes sore or other vaginal problem is present, this should not be done until the problem has resolved.) She should wash her hands and clip her nails prior to the massage. In a private environment, she should sit, semireclining, and relax her flexed, opened legs. Using a vegetable oil or water-soluble lubricant, she will use her thumb or fingers to rub oil into the tissue between the vagina and the anus and into the first inch or two of the vagina. The urinary opening should be avoided. If performed by a partner, the index finger may be preferred.

With the thumb or fingers inside the vagina, she will press downward toward her anus and out toward her sides, maintaining gentle, firm pressure until she feels a slight stinging, tingling, or burning sensation. She should sustain this for about two minutes until numbness begins to occur in the area. Then she should maintain the pressure for another three to four minutes while she slowly strokes back and forth from the midline toward the sides of the vagina, simultaneously pulling down toward her anus.[52]

In addition to teaching perineal self-massage, a practitioner may perform specific techniques that release chronic tension and extinguish trigger points in the pelvic floor musculature and fascial tissues. Of course, these techniques would not be performed without the client's consent. With work in this most intimate area, respect must also be paid to the legal limitations for practitioners and to the woman's comfort level, both emotionally and physically. Use sensitive deep tissue compressions and tiny, fingertip kneading on the attachments along the medial pubic ramus to relax the transverse perineal and levator ani muscles. **Massage techniques performed internally by the practitioner are always contraindicated, even with the woman's consent or request.**

Flexibility and relaxation

*W*omen need flexibility in order to labor most efficiently and comfortably. She may want to labor in positions such as squatting, kneeling, and on all-fours that require even more leg and pelvic flexibility. To prepare her for labor, include appropriate deep tissue, stretches, assisted-resisted exercise, and other passive movements and techniques that reduce chronic tension and increase flexibility in the following areas: thigh adductors, quadriceps group, hamstring group, the lateral and medial rotators of the hip, the iliotibial tract, and the lumbar spine.

Most childbirth education classes teach several relaxation techniques that are beneficial during pregnancy and essential during labor, including progressive, active, and autogenic relaxation.[53] Some women enjoy practicing these techniques during body therapy sessions. Clients should practice breathing diaphragmatically, and they may even want to practice using the breath to remain relaxed during any more intense therapy procedures. Encourage regular relaxation times,

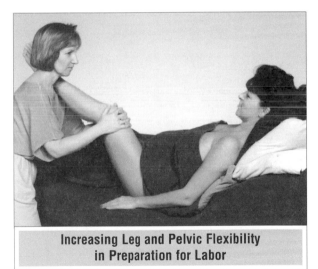

Increasing Leg and Pelvic Flexibility in Preparation for Labor

and enhance the client's relaxation capacity by either building on techniques already learned or by teaching other methods. Relaxation visualizations, touch relaxation (sensate focusing), and pregnancy yoga are techniques that are highly compatible with body therapy sessions.[54, 55, 56]

Body therapy is, by its very nature, a lesson in relaxation. Practitioners can also deliberately empower pregnant clients with heightened physical and emotional skills for relaxation. Cultivate a demeanor, touch, and techniques that foster the client's internal awareness, kinesthetic learning, and her ability to let go.

♦ ♦ SENSATE FOCUSING ♦ ♦

Reduce the effects of stress and improve kinesthetic awareness and control of muscular tension levels by training clients to relax to focused touch. Include the following exercise in your sessions, and help partners learn to similarly facilitate relaxation, which is especially critical during labor.

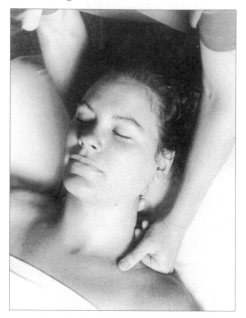

1. Beginning at the feet, head, or a client-designated area, slowly and methodically stroke superficially over her entire body.
2. At identified tension sites, stop to apply gentle pressure. Instruct her to inhale as though she were touching the tension with her breath and to exhale while imagining releasing the tension into your hands and with her breath.

♦ ♦ ♦ ♦

Partner's massage instruction

*M*assage instruction for partners is especially beneficial for reducing pregnancy discomforts and promoting communication between expectant couples. Techniques such as effleurage and kneading which do not require advanced anatomical knowledge or refined palpatory skills are appropriate to include in couples' pregnancy massage classes.[57] Couples appreciate knowing labor massage techniques, and infant massage instruction[58, 59, 60] can greatly benefit the growing family.

Post-term pregnancies

*D*espite measurements, testing, and proper prenatal and self-care, 3%-14% of women's pregnancies go beyond their calculated due dates. The causes of gestation beyond forty-two weeks are obscure; however, potential problems include decreased amniotic fluid, fetal fecal contamination of amniotic fluid, and placental and umbilical cord aging and malfunctioning. These conditions can result in large babies (macrosomia) and fetal physiological imbalances as well as maternal exhaustion, fear, and frustration.[61] Discomfort and impatience amplify any anxiety she feels, so more frequent relaxation massage is helpful. Once a woman is "overdue," she may request stimulation of reflexive hand, calf, and foot points contraindicated until now. Teach her how to work with these points, and encourage thrice daily, 5 to 10-minute self-massage periods. Encourage her to consider other non-pharmacological labor initiation techniques such as nipple stimulation by her or her partner, orgasm, or vigorous activities.[62]

Frequently she benefits from exploring her readiness for motherhood with gentle probes such as "What else do you need to feel ready for your baby?" "Are there any ways in which you are resisting or reluctant to birth?" "What are your fears or concerns?"

Summary of recommended third trimester bodywork

In the twenty-seventh week through term, pregnant women will benefit from these therapeutic somatic activities:

- ♦ **Body-use education** in diaphragmatic breathing and in increased posterior and lateral-costal breathing capacity; pelvic tilting and iliopsoas development; postural alignment and body usage instruction; appropriate abdominal strengthening activities, with modifications for diastus recti; strengthening, relaxation, and awareness of the pelvic floor musculature, especially by Kegel exercises.
- ♦ **Cross-fiber, deep tissue, lomi-lomi, positional release, passive movement, stretching, structural balancing, trigger point, and connective tissue massage techniques** to reduce strain on the joints, especially the sacroiliac, lumbosacral, symphysis pubis, hips, rib cage, and scapulothoracic joints. The soft tissues of these areas, particularly superficial back fascial line and lumbodorsal fascia, erector spinae, intrinsic spinal extensors and rotators, hip rotators, trapezius, levator scapulae, supraspinatus, pectoralis major, and pectoralis minor muscles also require attention.
- ♦ **Preparation for birthing** by deep tissue, myofascial, passive movement, and trigger point techniques to release chronic tension and increase flexibility in the adductors, quadriceps, hamstrings, and rotators of the hip joint so that she may more comfortably assume a variety of

positions during labor.

♦ **Preparation of the pelvic floor for birth** by Kegel exercises and perineal self-massage instruction, as well as appropriate deep tissue work to the pubic attachments of the pelvic floor musculature.

♦ **Teaching partners appropriate massage and relaxation techniques** to enhance the family's ability to support the laboring woman as she gives birth.

♦ **Myofascial, stretching, postural alignment, and support measures** to relieve pain from strain to all of the ligaments of the uterus, as it supports the tremendous growth of the baby in this trimester.

♦ **Swedish, lymphatic drainage, craniosacral, and reflexive techniques** to assist in circulation, to reduce stress and fatigue, relieve constipation, hemorrhoids, heartburn, and other complaints, and to facilitate general physiological processes.

♦ **Swedish, stretching, connective tissue, and appropriate deep tissue work** to assist in preventing and/or relieving edema in the feet and legs, varicose veins, cramps in the gastrocnemius/soleus and peroneal muscles, and "restless legs."

♦ **Nurturing, gentle, touch** to reduce stress and create a supportive, caring experience.

♦ **Nonjudgmental, active listening** that assists her in processing feelings and emotional issues. Be especially alert to concerns about body image, sexual activity, spousal or sexual abuse issues, her health and/or the baby's development, changes in relationships, dependence, previous problematic pregnancies, anxieties about the impending labor and birth, and other emotional issues she may be experiencing. Provide appropriate referrals to other professionals as needed.

♦ **Experiences of deep relaxation, internal focus, and awareness,** through touch, visualizations, and other autogenic relaxation techniques, emphasizing relaxing through intense stimulus and pain, as she will need to do in labor.

♦ **Instruction in infant massage and movement routines** to encourage the bonding and well-being of the newborn and its family.

"Sandy began coming for treatment in the fifth month of her second pregnancy. The birth of her daughter Emily had been long and arduous with back labour, and Sandy was starting to experience back pain, sciatic like pain down her leg, and increasing anxiety about the pending labour. At her sessions we worked together on progressive relaxation and breathing as a strong base for labour preparation, on keeping free the hard working parascapular musculature heavily used in caring for her one-year-old daughter, and lots of attention to her sacral and hip area.

A regular routine of deep tissue work to the sacral ligaments, the attachments above and below the iliac crest, and especially releasing the piriformis were exactly what Sandy needed to alleviate her pain and then, slowly gain confidence that this labour would and could be different. She continued to come for treatment every two weeks until the last month, then weekly until her second daughter was born. I remember picking up her laughing message telling me she had given birth to Hayley three hours before after five hours of manageable rhythmic labour, no back pain, and just three pushes!

It is my experience – the shared experience of many, many moms-to-be — that working with the hip and sacral regions are "magic" for the expectant mom and always effective in freeing up movement and reducing, if not eliminating, low back, sacral, and gluteal pain." — Linda Hickey, registered massage therapist, Calgary, Alberta, Canada

"One of my clients had an unexpected pregnancy a few years after [she turned] 40. This woman was a physical therapist, and, though she had helped many people deal with chronic pain, she had never experienced it herself. As she moved into the second trimester of pregnancy, she began waking up at night with fiery, electric pain in both arms and hands. Her obstetrician diagnosed pregnancy-related carpal tunnel syndrome. Informing this very active woman that her last ultrasound had revealed a potentially dangerous condition called placenta previa, he put her on bed rest.

When she came to see me she was quite upset about how things were unfolding, and was concerned that the carpal tunnel would last beyond pregnancy. We began our session with circulatory work in the hands and arms, and she was relieved to find that her pain diminished dramatically. We both agreed that the pain was more likely due to fluid in the arms than a structural discrepancy. In subsequent sessions, when I was traveling to her house, we spent some time instructing her husband in the art of Swedish arm massage so that he would be able to offer her some relief during the time in between sessions. Her carpal tunnel discontinued when she finished breastfeeding." — Liz Ellis, massage therapist, Chicago, IL

"A client was referred to me by her obstetrician because of severe low back pain. She believes that her back had been out of alignment since her previous pregnancy five years earlier when she gained over 60 pounds and was confined to bed with pre-term labor. She delivered her first child, a son, at 35 weeks after breaking through medication to prevent preterm labor.

As I evaluated her structural alignment, I discovered that her L3 was extremely anterior and her L4 was equally posterior. The therapy we created for her consisted of exercises to tone both right and left psoas muscles and massage work to relax, stretch, and restore proper blood flow to all the muscles of the low back and hip girdle. This therapy allowed her to stay physically active much farther into her pregnancy than the first time.

She again had pre-term labor problems, but with massage therapy we were able to keep her catecholamines at a low level. These are the hormones that build up when the body can neither flee nor fight when confronted with stress. Together with her more relaxed state of mind and terbutaline medication, she was able to maintain her pregnancy through the thirty-seventh week before delivering her second son.

Her postpartum recovery was much easier because we were able to strengthen her low back, plus she had gained only 35 pounds. She felt totally supported both emotionally and physically throughout her pregnancy by massage."

— Carroll Patterson, registered massage therapist, Austin, TX

Chapter

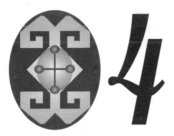

4

Labor and Birth Facilitation

Birthing is one of the most profound experiences in life; an inspirational voyage of courage, endurance, pain, and ecstasy. As part of a team of perinatal professionals, the somatic practitioner may accompany a woman on that journey as an active caregiver. Understanding the physiological and emotional dynamics of labor and birth prepares the practitioner to offer consistent emotional and tactile nurturance to the laboring woman. As the primary facilitator of relaxation, energy conservation and regeneration, pain management, and labor facilitation, practitioners may enhance the birth experience. This chapter provides an overview of labor and birth, including vital guidance for assisting the laboring woman, and sidebars detailing the most essential labor techniques.

An Overview of Labor

*A*fter months of fostering the optimal environment for the growth and nurturance of the fetus, endocrine alterations occur in both the mother and the fetus. These changes cause the uterine muscular fibers to practice their first mild, uncoordinated contractions. The pregnant woman may not even notice these pre-labor contractions (Braxton-Hicks contractions), but they begin the process of softening, shortening, thinning, and opening the cervix. In later pregnancy these contractions become stronger and more rhythmic, leading to the perception that labor has begun. If a change of activities stops them, she has been experiencing "false labor."

As labor approaches, the baby's head may naturally "engage," sinking firmly against the cervix. This "dropping" or "lightening" will help the expectant woman breathe more easily and reduce heartburn and digestive discomforts, but she will urinate more frequently because the baby's head is compressing her bladder. Muscular and ligament pain in her back and pelvis often become more severe as relaxin levels elevate and the baby grows. Vaginal secretions increase, and her breasts produce more colostrum, the baby's first food after birth.

Several days or hours prior to labor, the mucus plug loosens from the gradually ripening cervix, usually evidenced by a bloodstained or dark discharge. A trickle or a gush of amniotic fluid from her vagina may signal the breaking of the uterine amniotic sac in which the baby has been floating, although amniotic membranes may not rupture until after labor begins.

During labor a progression of contractions of three layers of uterine muscles alters the uterus to allow the baby's passage through the cervix and down the

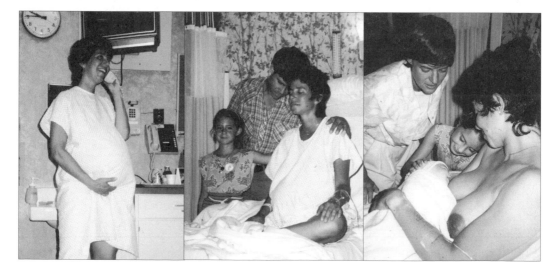

vagina to its birth. Labor is an intricately fascinating orchestration of endocrine activity and autonomic nervous system coordination which creates these structural changes to the uterus. Labor alters brain functions and creates deep levels of psychological and spiritual stimulation. It is both a transition from in utero to external life for the baby, and it is a passage into motherhood for the pregnant woman.

Pregnant women generally greet the onset of labor with relief and eager anticipation; many also feel uncertain, anxious, and unprepared if labor begins before the due date. If past due, she may feel quite frustrated and distracted. In the first stage of labor, contractions of the vertical uterine muscle fibers thin the closed, tube-shaped cervix (effacement) and open it (dilation) to 10 centimeters wide.

This relatively long stage is followed by a second stage when the diagonal and horizontal uterine muscle layers squeeze and press the baby through the dilated cervix, down the vaginal tunnel (birth canal), and out into the world. The one to two hours of strenuous work in second stage labor are usually a tremendously joyous relief, and many women and their partners are energized by the imminence of their baby's birth. First time mothers may also be somewhat frightened by the overwhelming, primitive urge to push, and may be fearful of perineal tearing. The climax of second stage labor is, obviously, the ecstatic moment of the birth of the baby as he slides out of her vagina. Although the strongest uterine contractions occur in the final, third stage, most women are relatively unaware of the expulsion of the placenta shortly after the birth.

LABOR MASSAGE THERAPY

*P*repare for your role at your client's labor by clarifying her expectations of you, and ask her to share any birth plan that she may have designed. Discuss how you may facilitate her labor with physical and emotional support. Invite her to share any painful, emotional previous experiences which may impact the birth. From this, you may learn how she tends to respond to pain and what has been helpful to her in the past. Assemble your equipment. Organize your professional and personal life to be ready for her, and be sure you have directions to her home or hospital. Develop a reliable communication system so that she feels assured of your availability.

Women respond with wide variation to touch and massage therapy during labor. Some may prefer to be undisturbed during part or all of their labors. Some cope best when massaged during contractions, and others only appreciate contact between contractions. Some require constant cutaneous stimulation to meet their physical and emotional needs. Many only want certain types of strokes, pressures, or rhythms, or respond best to only specific areas being massaged. During contractions, slow, rhythmic, predictable movements are generally best; stationary compressions also are effective. Often a woman's preferences change greatly over the hours of her labor. Effectiveness of techniques also varies greatly with different women and in different labor stages. If a particular technique is not successful in early first stage labor, experiment later to test its effectiveness. Be flexible about abandoning techniques that become ineffective. Experiment and improvise generously.

Remember that a laboring woman is still pregnant. Continue to observe contraindications regarding types of techniques and their applications as described in Chapter Two; however, you may now press the uterine zones and acupuncture points to stimulate labor. Be particularly cautious in working on her legs as her blood becomes even more likely to clot (hypercoagulable) perinatally.

General Guidelines For Labor Massage

During Contractions:	Between Contractions:
Slow, firm, predictable strokes	Flush lactic acid
Stationary compression	Stretching
Rhythmic movement	Positional changes

Observe all prenatal contraindications and precautions, except contraction stimulation points.

EARLY FIRST STAGE LABOR

*O*nce uterine contractions reach sufficient intensity, duration, and sustained regularity to begin to dilate the cervix (generally 5-8 minutes between contractions), first stage labor has begun. This latent stage includes effacement and dilation of the cervix to a three-centimeter opening. It is generally the longest stage and lasts between 12 and 14 hours, but it may extend for more than a day, especially for first-time mothers.

In the early phase, the laboring woman may feel low, nagging backache and menstrual-like cramps that become increasingly painful. How she responds to these intensifying contractions significantly determines the progress of her labor. Although the baby's hypothalamus, pituitary, and adrenal glands initiated labor, the mother's endocrine and autonomic nervous system govern its progress.[1] Sympathetic and parasympathetic nerves of the autonomic nervous system enervate the uterine smooth muscle layers. The labor hormones, norepinephrine and epinephrine, stimulate uterine muscle contractions. A relaxed woman's parasympathetic arousal contributes to balanced hormone levels, and the improved ability of the uterine muscle cell receptors to pick up and to respond to hormonal signals.[2] With parasympathetic stimulation, or relaxation, the circular fibers relax so that

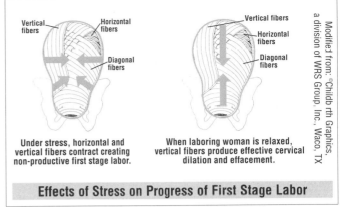

Under stress, horizontal and vertical fibers contract creating non-productive first stage labor.

When laboring woman is relaxed, vertical fibers produce effective cervical dilation and effacement.

Modified from: ©Childbirth Graphics, a division of WRS Group, Inc., Waco, TX

Effects of Stress on Progress of First Stage Labor

effacement and dilation can proceed. Her labor progresses with strong, rhythmic, and effective contractions of the vertical uterine muscles.[3]

♦ ♦ FULL BODY SWEDISH OR ESALEN-STYLE MASSAGE THERAPY: ♦ ♦

Many laboring women enjoy a relaxing massage during early first stage labor. Often a complete therapeutic massage will help her to identify the individualized ways in which she responds to her contractions. Depending upon the amount of time between contractions, a one hour session provides eight or more opportunities to locate and relax tightening muscles, establish relaxation breathing, and explore coping strategies before active labor intensifies. She may be especially responsive to a guided visualization of the birth after a relaxing massage. Work with her at your office, her home, her hospital, or the birthing center.

♦ ♦ ♦ ♦

♦ ♦ RELAXING TENSE MUSCLES ♦ ♦

Most women respond to pain with some degree of generalized muscular tension. The most commonly tensed muscles during labor are: masseter and temporalis; trapezius, levator scapulae, and other upper back muscles; hand and finger flexors; hamstrings and quadriceps; adductor longus, brevis, and magnus; erector spinae, quadratus lumborum, and other lumbar muscles; levator ani, transverse perineal, and other pelvic floor muscles; gastrocnemius, soleus, and toe flexors.

1. Dissipate unproductive tension in these muscles with sensate focusing techniques. (See labor preparation, Chapter 3.)
2. During contractions, apply firm, stationary, deep tissue compressions with knuckles, fist, fingers, or elbow. Cause no pain, and maintain

consistency of touch. (See second trimester techniques, Chapter 3.)

3. Kneading, effleurage, and other Swedish strokes help to flush lactic acid from chronically tightened muscles and prevent cramping. Perform rhythmic, firm strokes during or between contractions, as she prefers. Between contractions also use passive stretches, assisted-resisted stretches, and/or shortening of tensed muscles to relax these areas by eliciting proprioceptive adjustments in muscle length.

♦ ♦ ♦ ♦

Despite the escalating intensity, in early labor many women can continue with normal activities, perhaps only pausing briefly to maintain relaxation and concentration as contractions peak. Most women spend part of their labor in their own homes. As some perinatal experts challenge the myth that a hospital is the safest place for all women to give birth, a small, but growing, number of North American women are choosing planned home births.[4, 5] Although she may transfer to a hospital or birthing center, you may begin supporting her labor at her home for several hours, or the whole day. During this latency period, she also may doze, take a walk or a shower, call friends and family, and lounge and cuddle with her partner. She may be excited, anticipatory, or nervous.

Anxiety stimulates sympathetic arousal, which overstimulates production of both labor hormones, resulting in slow, ineffectual, painful labor. Sympathetic stimulation negatively affects first stage labor by creating contractions in the layer of horizontal, circular fibers that comprises most of the cervix so that the anxious woman's cervix tightens against vertical muscle contractions intended to open it. (See illustration, previous page.) Blood flow to the uterus also is reduced by as much as 65%.[6]

First stage labor proceeds best when a woman relaxes, letting her uterus work with no interference from mental or physical tension. She may soothe herself with rhythmic movements such as walking, swaying, dancing, rocking, and deep abdominal breathing. (See diaphragmatic breathing, Chapter 3.) She may develop visualizations or rituals that create a predictable pattern or sequence of coping activities. Attentive, nurturing presence and touch from her family, friends, and you may comfort her immensely. Calm her, and reassure her that her pain is, as Sheila Kitzinger describes it, "pain with a purpose."[7] Anyone who has attempted to calm a frightened child knows that relaxation is far easier to maintain than to recover. Maximize relaxation early in labor to help ensure parasympathetic arousal as labor intensifies. Encourage her to change positions frequently, usually every 20-30 minutes, and, when possible, to maximize gravity's assistance by standing, squatting, or sitting. Remind her to regularly empty her bladder.

♦ ♦ MINI-MASSAGES ♦ ♦

Some women relax best to massage therapy in only one or two areas, particularly their face, hands, feet or abdomen.

1. Experiment with gentle, soothing facial massage, especially to the scalp, forehead, and jaw. Hair stroking is very nurturing for many. Include her neck and upper shoulders. Gently undulate her cervical spine, and the atlanto-occipital joint.

2. Thoroughly massage both of her hands, especially if she has been clenching them during contractions. Firm, midline palmar pressure simultaneous with friction on the dorsal surface of her hand simulates a traditional labor technique of clenching a comb or other object without generating forearm tension. Simkin theorizes that this technique's effectiveness is due to the abundance of pressure sensors (Pacinian corpules) in the palm.[8] Stimulate the Hoku point in the posterior webbing between her thumb and index finger, deep in the proximal joint to promote vigorous contractions.

3. Use Swedish, passive movements, or reflexive work on her feet. Apply firm, rhythmic inching pressure to create bone-to-bone contact at the zones reflexive to areas of tension and pain. Concentrate on the pelvic, perineal, and back reflexes. To encourage contractions, press the uterine points on the medial calcaneus, described in Chapter Two, and the acupuncture points illustrated later in this chapter.

4. Encourage relaxation by performing a gentle, superficial effleurage of her abdomen, or teaching the strokes to the laboring woman or her partner. Use long strokes and circular fingertip movements that flow upward from the pubic area to simulate the lifting force of the uterine muscles on the dilating and effacing cervix. Amplify this effect by suggesting that she visualize each contraction gathering the cervix into the uterine walls to open it. When the belt of an electronic fetal monitor restricts long strokes, shorten your strokes, and emphasize rhythm and purpose of the stroke.

♦ ♦ ♦ ♦

♦ ♦ CRANIOSACRAL THERAPY ♦ ♦

Craniosacral therapy fosters relaxation and balance in all body systems. It is particularly useful during labor for maintaining physiologic equilibrium (homeostasis).

1. Induce stillpoint of the craniosacral fluid rhythms by holding then releasing the ebbing and flowing fluid with light pressure against the mastoid area of the temporal bones; through holding the legs; or at the sacrum.

2. Follow with release of the occipital cranial base, the thoracic inlet, and the pelvic and respiratory diaphragms.

3. Relieve pelvic pain with sacral compression/decompression techniques. Use the V-spread to focus healing energy at specific painful areas.

♦ ♦ ♦ ♦

ACTIVE FIRST STAGE LABOR

As first stage labor moves into its active phase, the contractions will become more intense, longer, and more frequent (30-45 seconds long, every 2-3 minutes). The cervix will continue to thin and open, achieving seven centimeters of dilation by this phase's end. With first-time mothers, this stage generally lasts between two and six hours. While some women experience very little pain, most will need to actively concentrate on optimizing relaxation, particularly at the peak of contractions. Her initial excitement and anticipation may have evolved into focus and hard work by this point.

Some childbirth educators counsel women to interpret their experience of uterine contractions as "intense" rather than "painful"; however, most women are in pain during some or all of labor and birth. They feel pain in the uterus, cervix, vagina, perineum, abdomen, lumbar area, pelvis, hips, and thighs. Abdominal pain is caused by lack of oxygen (hypoxia) and increased lactic acid in the uterine muscles. As the cervix dilates, painful stretching of the lower uterus occurs. The engaged fetal head presses uncomfortably on adjacent structures, especially the low back, sacrum, symphysis pubis, and lumbosacral plexus. Contractions stretch and traction the uterine and pelvic ligaments. As the baby descends deeper into the pelvic outlet, it distends the vagina and perineum. Many women are emotionally very tense, resulting in generalized muscular tension.[9] Another pain source may be myofascial trigger points, particularly in the abdomen, paravertebral and perineal muscles, and muscles and ligaments in spasm or strained by the pregnancy. When musculoskeletal pain levels are high, uterine pain is more severe.

Fear, feeling alone, and other emotions and belief structures may cause as much pain during labor as contraction intensity and fetal size and position.[10] Women who have suffered sexual abuse are particularly vulnerable to negative emotional states. Procedures such as pelvic exams and injections can be experienced as violations. Exposure, fear of injury, and actual injury of sexual body parts increase her vulnerability and may evoke conscious or unconscious memories. She may struggle with control issues involved with surrendering to labor and trusting medical authorities.[11] For all women, exhaustion, nausea, and other physiological responses often aggravate anxiety, churning up a maelstrom of escalating pain and fear.

> *"I recently worked with a repeat client who had experienced a previous traumatic postpartum recovery from severe perineal and rectal tears. One of the concerns that I focused on during our pregnancy massage sessions was her fear of repeating her previous problems. I encouraged her to share her fears with her new obstetrician.*
>
> *Her labor was uneventful in the early stages. By the time she realized that she was in active labor, she had checked into the alternative birthing center, was dilated to six centimeters, and 100% effaced. Her husband used sacral compression and patterned her breathing while I used massage to help her focus on relaxing. She successfully birthed her 9 lb, 8 oz daughter an hour and a half later. She had a superficial tear, and the baby did experience a broken collar bone, but she was alert, making fantastic eye contact with her parents, and was a wonderful breastfeeder. The mother cannot believe how easy this postpartum recovery has been for her."* — Carroll Patterson, registered massage therapist, Austin, Texas

Preparation through childbirth classes usually helps a woman to cope productively with labor pain.[12] Women have many choices in childbirth philosophies including Bradley,[13] Lamaze,[14] Psychosexual,[15] and non-methodological or integrated preparation classes. With active participation in a class, she becomes more knowledgeable about labor. She is usually less fearful because she understands its progression, the sources of her pain, and she also is more skilled in coping and comfort strategies.

Of course the amount of pain she experiences and her ability to respond positively to that pain is influenced by many other factors including: ethnic and cultural beliefs and mores; her psychological make-up; intensity and frequency of contractions; fetal size and position; and the obstetrical interventions performed.[16] A woman's response to her labor experience is highly individualized. Some women labor using only non-pharmacological pain relief techniques such as those discussed in this chapter. Many use massage, movement,

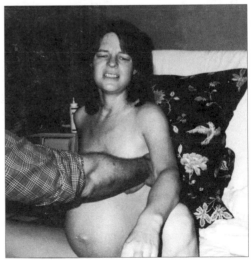

and other emotional and physical support to delay and reduce their use of pain medications. In her book, *Easing Labor Pain*, veteran childbirth educator, Adrianne Lieberman describes the use of transcutaneous electrical nerve stimulation (TENS), acupuncture, biofeedback, and hypnosis for pain management.[17] Others prefer a totally pain-free experience, relying on analgesia such as Demerol or codeine for pain relief, or anesthesia such as pentobarbital to create a loss of sensation. Author and doula Penny Simkin has created a very useful scale to help women determine their preferences in this regard. (See Resources appendix.)

Modern technology and medications are frequently touted as the answer to a laboring woman's prayers. While pharmacological pain reduction is usually effective and may be very beneficial, women are often unaware of its possible negative effects.[18, 19, 20] For example, epidural use is very popular in North America. With an epidural (continuous drip of analgesia into the epidural space of the spine), other interventions may become necessary such as Pitocin to stimulate a stalled labor, and forceps or vacuum extraction (instrument applied to the fetal head to assist in moving the baby down the vagina) to assist with diminished pushing sensations.[21] Epidural analgesia administered in early labor doubles or triples the likelihood of a cesarean birth.[22] Additionally, some research indicates that infants whose mothers had epidurals are less alert, less oriented, and less mature in motor skills during their first months than those whose mothers were unmedicated.[23] There is little research data available that measures the long term effect of epidural anesthesia on the infant or the mother.[24]

If she chooses or needs an epidural, she is usually bedridden. This may cause her to feel "sick," particularly if other interventions are then required. "Shot glass" or "walking epidurals" of reduced anesthesia are sometimes administered. The numbness she experiences from her waist down provides welcome pain relief; unfortunately some women then feel dissociated from their birth experience. Encourage her to massage her abdomen, allowing her hands to monitor the regularity and power of her contractions. She can minimize the negative circulatory effects of reduced activity by changing positions every 20 minutes when possible. If she must stay on one side, the upper side may have unanesthetized patches while circulation to the bottom leg is reduced. Perform thorough Swedish and lymphatic drainage to her legs and foot reflexology to increase and normalize circulation. Lateral recumbancy on a Contoured bodyCushion® or with sufficient pillows, as described in Chapter Three, may also help in normalizing circulation and in preventing shoulder compression and discomfort.

Modify your work to avoid disturbing the electronic fetal monitor that will be in place during an epidural. An intravenous drip (IV) will usually accompany an epidural, and it too must be avoided when working on her arms. Because many women sleep or may no longer need to work with their contractions, you may feel as though your support is superfluous; regardless of her pain level, most women continue to need emotional support and caring touch. During pushing you will be indispensable, as the anesthesia will make her unable to control her legs.

> *"I loved being pregnant, and felt prepared for a positive birth experience: a loving and supportive husband, childbirth education, a detailed birth plan, and an awesome supporting cast of my mother, my friend, Grace who is also my massage therapist, and another friend, all with birthing experience. Then, overdue and with low amniotic fluid levels, a pitocin induction seemed necessary. The night before I meditated, danced, and prayed that the baby would come on his own, but he didn't. So I took several deep breaths and made the best of it.*
>
> *We successfully elevated the energy of the L&D room to create an environment more supportive of birthing and the first hours went by with ease as Grace massaged me. Later, jasmine oil, sacral pressure, and Mark's steady comforting energy got me to five centimeters in six hours, but I was sure I couldn't continue. Reminding myself that God is in the drugs too, I asked for a 'shotglass' epidural. This was just right to give me a little rest, but not so much so that I couldn't feel anything. I completed dilation in just another hour, then began pushing. Grace massaged my neck and jaw, mom prayed and took photos, and my husband caught Bryce, after only four pushes. His birth is without a doubt the most significant ritual passage of my life, and my heart is forever expanded."* — Krishna

Some women feel strongly that a completely natural birth is critical to self-fulfillment as well as to avoid the negative effects of drugs on their baby and their labor. Fortunately, non-pharmacological pain relief has proven to be effective, especially when a woman has a reasonably normal labor. These "natural" coping strategies, such as movement, position changes, relaxation, breathing, massage therapy, and emotional support have few negative side effects.[25]

Simkin postulates that the efficacy of massage therapy and other types of comfort measures is explainable by the Gate Theory of Pain Control.[26] Sensory perception begins when the dorsal horn of the spinal cord receives impulses from the rest of the body via the afferent sensory nerves. Here they are transmitted to the brain for interpretation and response. Pleasurable, painful, and neutral signals travel on variously-sized afferent nerve fibers at different speeds, with pain traveling most slowly. According to Gate theorists Wall and Melzac, if the brain's receptor sites are filled by pressure, stroking, friction, heat, or cold, perception is closed, much like a gate, to any slower moving pain signals.[27] Pain management with these stimuli is most effective when continuous, varied tactile experiences are utilized during painful contractions.

In *Gentle Birth Choices*, Barbara Harper, R.N., reminds us of the role of endorphins, the body's natural painkillers and tranquilizers: "The levels of endorphins…increase during pregnancy reaching a peak during labor. As the body responds to the natural oxytocin that causes the uterus to contract, more endorphins are released into the system, reducing the pain and creating a sense of well-being. Runners describe a similar response in long-distance running, which they refer to as a 'runner's high'."[28]

♦ ♦ CONTRACTION DISTRACTION ♦ ♦

Flooding the brain with pleasurable sensations provides distraction from pain. You can help override pain signals emanating from the uterus by using pressure, pleasurable strokes, and passive movement stimuli to directly compete with painful contraction stimuli. The T10 to lumbosacral junction are the most effective areas to massage.

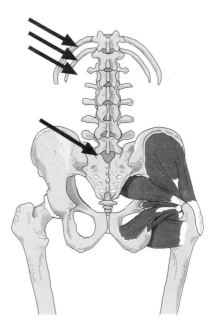

1. Use fingertips, thumbs, knuckles, or elbows to compress firmly and directly perpendicular to the paravertebral muscles at the level of T10 to L2. Apply this deep pressure into the lateral borders of the erector spinae, and also at the lumbosacral junction during contractions to compete with uterine sensations.
2. Perform rhythmic effleurage, kneading, thumb fanning, and/or nerve strokes to the area and to the entire sacrum during contractions.
3. Encourage rhythmic pelvic tilting during contractions.

4. Provide more general distraction with gentle abdominal effleurage; long, delicate strokes down the arms or legs; or soft, soothing fanning motions across the brow.

5. Reflexively address pain by stimulating Chinese acupuncture point, Bladder 67. During contractions, apply firm pressure bilaterally with a fingernail into the flesh at the lateral, proximal corner of the nails of the fifth toes.

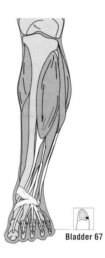

Bladder 67

◆ ◆ ◆ ◆

Changes in hemispheric brain functioning during labor further explain the potency of massage therapy and bodywork as labor support. In *Mind Over Labor*, Carl Jones calls these changes "the laboring mind response." During labor the brain gradually switches from a logical, rational, left hemisphere orientation, from which most operate in their daily lives. The intuitive, instinctual, creative right hemisphere becomes more active during labor. As a result, the laboring woman becomes so focused on her inner world that her time and space perceptions may become distorted. This also lowers her inhibitions so that she has less concern about the distinctly sexual positions, movements, expressions, and sounds that she may experience.[29]

Paradoxically, she simultaneously becomes more sensitive to those around her and to her environment. Being more open to mental suggestion in this state, she is both negatively influenced by seemingly minor remarks by those around her and positively affected by appropriate encouragement, images, and visualizations given to her. She may focus well on textured fabrics or photographs with repeating patterns, water, or other natural images of opening and power.[30] Creative, active imagery, positive statements (affirmations), and prayer are usually dynamically effective during labor.[31] Under right hemisphere influence, the laboring body is especially responsive to the messages of empathetic, therapeutic touch. The right brain magnifies the many nuances of appropriate touch so that a laboring woman will more strongly receive your tactile communications of nurturance, support, and strength.

Laboring Mind Response from *Mind Over Labor* by Carl Jones

♦ Right hemisphere brain orientation

♦ Internal orientation

♦ Heightened emotional and perceptual sensitivity

♦ Increased suggestibility

♦ Decreased inhibitions

♦ Distinctly sexual behavior

Labor's heightened physical and emotional state can be a rich environment for a woman's personal growth. Meeting labor's challenges and receiving respectful, empathetic care builds a good self-image, or may repair a poor self-image. Even long, complicated labors are satisfying experiences when a woman feels respected, cared for, and in control of decisions regarding her and her baby's care.[32] There is equal potential for damaging her self-esteem. Every birth has the potential to traumatize or retraumatize a woman. Labor can also increase her confidence, self-worth, and psychological health. Your nurturing presence during labor is potent in facilitating this type of empowering childbirth experience.

Ninety-five percent of women, when allowed to choose their most comfortable laboring positions, prefer being vertical. Contractions are more effective and intense when she is standing, walking, or sitting upright than when she is lying down. Upright positions tend to shorten the length of first stage labor by one-third, partially because this position maximizes gravity's positive effect on the birthing process. Vertical positions also minimize the risks of decreased fetal oxygen supply by taking pressure off of the maternal vena cava.[33]

Although squatting is particularly effective, many women are unable to assume a full squat for long. She may get similar effects by straddling a chair to open her thighs and pelvis, while resting her upper body against pillows propped on the chair back. Other alternatives include sitting on a toilet, kneeling in bed, or standing while supported by her partner. Be prepared to work with clients in a variety of positions. Encourage frequent changes of position, especially if labor stalls or slows. When labor progresses at an overwhelming speed or blood pressure rises, sidelying or semireclining positions may be required.

If she resists the increased emotional and physical intensity of active labor, muscular tension may become more problematic. When she develops tension in specific muscles during contractions, work with her as in early first stage labor. Encourage tiny, undulatory joint mobilizations (micromovements) of her hands, feet, or other tense areas. Relax generalized muscular tension with deep work on the posterior pelvis and on the intrinsic spinal musculature. Lumbar and pelvic pain from sacroiliac and lumbosacral joints often respond well to deep, specific strokes to the area, to stretching, and to other rhythmic, small amplitude passive movements. (See third trimester tech-

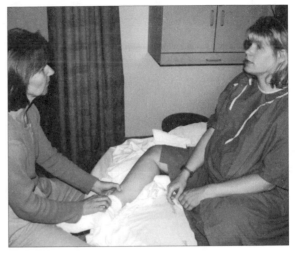

niques, Chapter 3.) Many of the techniques detailed in the previous section on early first stage labor also will be appropriate in active first stage labor.

Careful use of heat and/or cold applications may also reduce pain, soothe the mother, or stimulate labor.[34] Cold packs are most helpful with musculoskeletal and joint pain, especially in the lumbar and pelvic areas. Warm baths or showers and heated blankets are relaxing and com-

forting for many. When a woman is in active labor, extended immersion in warm tubs (98°-100° F) slows escalating pain, improves cervical dilation, reduces augmentation interventions, and increases her satisfaction with her labor.[35] Many other potential benefits include reduced blood pressure, lower incidence and severity of perineal tearing and the need for episiotomies, and easier adjustment for the newborn.[36] Careful application of heat over the upper uterine area has been shown to increase uterine activity without risks to the fetus.[37]

Recent observations of maternity nurses' activities revealed only two instances of reassuring touch out of 616 interactions with laboring women. When they touched women, they were primarily attending to clinical tasks such as pulse reading, vaginal exams, and securing equipment. Less than 10% of all their activities were emotionally supportive in any way.[38] Many nurses are very dissatisfied with this change in activities from primarily a nurturing role to an equipment monitor role. In a "high tech" environment, the balancing effects of "high touch" are generally appreciated.

While a somatic practitioner can be a valuable addition to a birthing group, she is in no way a replacement for labor and delivery nurses, nor for trained mid-wives, nurse-midwives, or physicians. Clearly identify yourself to the attending perinatal team, and function within your scope of practice. Stay current with their profile of the labor's status, including pelvic station, dilation, and fetal position, but remember you are not responsible for such monitoring. While you may be one of her advocates, you are not her "coach" unless she has designated you so. Your presence should not supplant a partner's care, but rather should enhance his or her focus on loving, attentive nurturing that deepens their birthing experience. Suggest appropriate touch and support to her attending family or friends when they seek your guidance. Remember that your primary role at a birth will be to facilitate relaxation, reduce pain and muscle cramping, and bolster energy levels.

When first stage labors are slow and painful, but not productive (protracted or prodromal labor), various massage therapy interventions may be helpful. First, reduce sympathetic nervous system arousal with relaxing centering touch employing rhythmic, soothing strokes. Using zone therapy to the entire foot, pressing deeply into the uterus points on the medial calcaneus is often effective. Craniosacral therapy and empathetic encouragement may also help. Unless she requests otherwise, maintain close, supportive physical contact with the mother, or have her partner do so. Try out a variety of gravity-assisted positions, walking, bathing or showering, and rhythmic activities.

♦ ♦ LABOR STIMULATION POINTS ♦ ♦

Certain Chinese acupuncture points can initiate and stimulate uterine contractions. In lieu of acupuncture needles, press firmly with thumbtip or fingertip bilaterally into the following points: Liver 3, Kidney 3, and Spleen 6. (These same points are contraindicated prior to a woman's due date.)

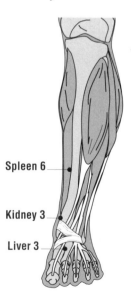

1. Liver 3 is located dorsally at the proximal junction of the first and second metatarsal bones of the foot.
2. Kidney 3 is on the superior border and just posterior to the medial malleolus of the ankle when the foot is held in dorsi-flexion.
3. Spleen 6 is located just posterior to the medial edge of the tibia, four client finger widths proximal to the medial malleolus (or 5/16's of the distance from the medial malleolus to the crease of the knee).
4. Work in six cycles of 10 seconds of pressure on and 10 seconds off. If not effective, extend your pressure to as long as one minute on and one minute off.

Spleen 6

Kidney 3

Liver 3

♦ ♦ ♦ ♦

♦ ♦ CERVICAL AND PELVIC FLOOR RELAXATION ♦ ♦

A relaxed cervix is more readily dilated by contractions. When the pelvic floor remains relaxed, the laboring woman yields to the power of contractions rather than resisting them. Relaxation of the pelvic floor appears to be closely related to relaxation of the jaw and mouth.[39]

1. Encourage open mouth exhalations to prevent her from clenching her jaws in response to the pain.
2. Validate and support any low-pitched, guttural vocalizations she makes such as groaning, moaning, and repeated sounds. If her vocalizations become high pitched and strident, she may be expressing fear, and she'll be tighter in her upper body. Use your own voice to lead her to lower sounds that will calm her, bring her awareness deeper into her belly, relax her throat, and help to keep the masseter and temporalis muscles relaxed.
3. Use imagery and visualizations to assist in opening of the cervix and relaxation of the pelvic floor muscles. For example, ask her to imagine that her cervix is the bud of her favorite flower. As each contraction begins and peaks, encourage her to imagine the bud slowly and easily opening into a large beautiful blossom, adding as much sensorial detail as possible.[40]
4. Also see toe press, second stage labor.

————— ♦ ♦ ♦ ♦ —————

Backache in Labor

One quarter to two thirds of women experience intense lumbar and sacral pain during labor.[41] This back labor is more prevalent if the baby is not optimally positioned with its head down, facing the mother's sacrum (anterior presentation or occiput anterior, OA). In the posterior presentation (occiput posterior or OP), the baby faces the mother's navel, its occiput against her lower spine and sacrum. In addition to not fitting as easily into the pelvis, this results in the baby's head creating more painful pressure on the sacral nerves and other pelvic structures, particularly straining the SI joint ligaments. Fortunately most OP babies rotate spontaneously during labor, and the severe back pain subsides.

Encourage persistent OP babies to rotate by supporting the woman as she tries walking, rocking or rotating her pelvis, or kneeling on pillows or in the bed. Lying on her side with her knees as close to her chest as possible for 30-45 minutes, or pelvic tilting while lifting the abdomen often allows the baby more room in which to rotate and can make contractions more regular and effective.[42] Avoid semireclining position for extended periods. Suggest changing position two to three times an hour. If her nurse or midwife can identify where the baby is, firmly but gently stroke her abdomen laterally to medially to help shift the baby to a better position.[43] When a baby remains in the posterior presentation, labor is usually longer, more painful, and more likely to require interventions, including forceps or a cesarean section.

Heat or cold, shower water, or a vibrator applied to the sacrum also may be effective in sending competing stimuli to the brain. Also encourage her to try an "all fours" position on her hands and knees to facilitate pelvic tilting and rocking of her body forward then back. These movements, especially in combination with the sacral counterpressure or cold packs, are often effective in reducing or eliminating back labor. You also may want to experiment with Simkin's "double hip squeeze;" use both hands to compress diagonally toward the sacrum into the bellies of the gluteal muscles during contractions. She also suggests leaning against both knees of the seated mother, pressing her femurs into the acetabulum during contractions to open and relieve pain in the SI joint.[44]

♦ ♦ SACRAL COUNTERPRESSURE ♦ ♦

Very firm sacral pressure will offer back labor relief, especially if the specific sacral sulcus where a nerve is being affected is identified. Pointed pressure in this area also stimulates the acupuncture points that coincide with these sulcuses (Urinary Bladder 31-34) to stimulate contractions. Because very deep pressure is necessary to create sufficient counterpressure, use your elbow, knee, or knuckle in efficient structural alignment as you apply your body weight.

1. From a position behind the client, apply very deep compressions on the sacrum. Search for one or two specific points which, when firmly pressed, afford relief ("sweet spot"). Maintain firm pressure continuously during each contraction.

2. Do not press the lumbar spine anteriorly with your pressure. Protect her lumbar spine by simultaneously directing your pressure inferiorly toward her coccyx, creating a passive pelvic tilt. You may also wish to support her pelvis with your other hand.

3. Relocate further distally on her sacrum or switch to the other side of her sacrum to find a new "sweet spot" when relief begins to diminish because the baby has moved.

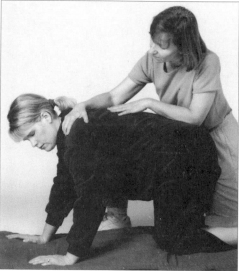

♦ ♦ ♦ ♦

TRANSITION PHASE OF FIRST STAGE

*O*ften the most emotionally and physically challenging phase of labor is transition. This brief phase includes the final effacement and dilation of the cervix from seven to a complete 10 centimeters. Transition contractions are typically long, painful, and frequent, often having no rest period between them. Earlier contractions tended to have rhythmic, smoothly sloped peaks of intensity. Contractions during transition may have many peaks of severe pain. They may seem to end, then shoot back up to peak intensity. Sometimes the cervix remains thickened, partially obstructing the baby's descent, yet expulsive contractions begin. This demanding, but premature urge to push with a cervical "lip" remaining can be especially difficult.

The mother also may experience wildly varying needs that change from moment to moment, including her desire for touch, assurance, warmth, and position changes. Nausea and vomiting are common during transition, as is leg and arm trembling. Feeling discouraged and exhausted from the previous efforts of the labor, women often declare that they are quitting, that they can take no more. Angry outbursts, crying, whimpering, groaning, or other emotional expressions are common. Many women find this phase very difficult to experience without tensing, fighting the process, or becoming physically and emotionally overwhelmed.

Particularly during contractions, avoid touch that is distracting to the laboring woman since she will likely need to concentrate on maintaining relaxation. Often a firm, still hand on an area of tension will be the only beneficial touch during a transition contraction. She may welcome slow, rhythmic massage or zone therapy on her feet. Backache is common, even with an anterior presentation baby, so concentrate on firm, deep pressure on her sacrum, SI joints, and paravertebral muscles. Firm, rhythmic effleurage moving proximal to distal on her inner thighs may help calm her trembling legs.

Steady eye contact often assures her of the presence of supportive companions and helps her to stay focused. She may find that a lighter, more rapid breathing pattern helps her to avoid premature pushing. Encourage her to meet the intensity of each contraction and to ride them one at a time. Guide her to stay "grounded," riding the swells of intensity rather than fighting them, through use of visualizations of powerful natural images such as ocean waves or waterfalls.[45] Reassure her that the intensity of this phase is a positive signal that labor has progressed significantly.

SECOND STAGE LABOR

*A*fter the tumultuous transition phase, second stage labor often begins with a resting phase. During this welcomed pause, the uterus imperceptibly shortens and tightens itself against the baby's torso, since the head has now moved into the vagina. While providing an opportunity to recharge herself, this phase is usually only 10-20 minutes long. Most women and their partners greet second stage labor with renewed energy and relief knowing that soon they will be able to hold their baby.

An undeniable urgency to bear down characterizes the descent phase of second stage labor. This urge to push is created by the pressure of the baby in the vagina and by contractions primarily of the circular and diagonally criss-crossed uterine muscle layers. With effacement and dilation complete, these muscles, assisted by the diaphragm, continue to push the baby down the vagina to its birth. The sensations of second stage contractions are different from those in the first stage. Not only are contractions closer to a minute in length and 3-5 minutes apart, but pushing contractions also have a plateau of intensity rather than a peak. The downward urgency occurs several times in each contraction, creating the most efficient times to bear down (spontaneous pushing).

While this is hard work, many women find the bearing down easier and much more satisfying than the more passive responses needed in first stage labor. While she must continue to conserve energy and relax as fully as possible, some exertion may be required. As she bears down in response to the urge to push, she may want to assist the uterine muscles with pressure from her abdomen and diaphragm. It is especially important that her pelvic floor and inner thighs remain relaxed so that tension here does not fight the baby's pressure from above.

Often the somatic practitioner's role also will change in second stage. The laboring woman may need you to support her leg or may wish to rest against you. Squatting women often need assistance in standing up between contractions. Should she feel no urge to push, she may want your guidance in when and how to bear down. Continue to focus, however, on relaxation, pain reduction, and energy conservation as discussed in previous sections.

Abdominal effleurage may be more effective in this phase when performed from the fundus down toward the pubis to match the expulsive forces of the contractions. Passive movements and visualizations are especially helpful in relaxing the adductor muscles. Between contractions, support the weight of her leg and rhythmically, gently rock the thigh between abduction and adduction movements. Indirectly relax the pelvic floor and inner thighs by gently squeezing together the big toe and next two toes of both feet. Hold or rhythmically release then hold these toes during contractions. Help her to keep her jaw and mouth relaxed.

Prolonged second stage labors usually require massage techniques that relieve exhaustion and cramping and assist the mother in maintaining a variety of positions. Swedish massage techniques and stretching of the muscles of flexed joints are critical between contractions. Squatting and other gravity-assisted positions may be more

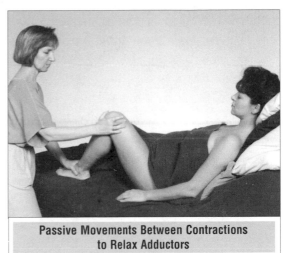

Passive Movements Between Contractions to Relax Adductors

achievable when the practitioner releases and stretches the hamstrings, adductors, and spinal musculature. The laboring woman may need additional positional support from the practitioner and others in order to conserve her energy for pushing, to open the pelvic outlet, and to assist the baby's movement down the birth canal. Back labor may continue or begin in this second stage, requiring deep sacral pressure and other measures as detailed in the section on active first stage labor. Immersion in warm water may be helpful.

♦ ♦ PELVIC PRESS ♦ ♦

Pressure applied to the lateral pelvis can mechanically increase the pelvic outlet by opening the symphysis pubis and sacral joints. This will allow the baby's head to descend more readily. The pelvic press is doubly effective when applied while the laboring woman also rocks herself forward and back during contractions.

1. Place your hands firmly on her iliac crests and press toward her midline evenly until you feel the motion of her pelvis. Hold your pressure during each contraction.
2. When she is on all fours or squatting, use a knee to press into one ilium, while reaching across her torso with your other hand to pull the other ilium toward your knee. Alternatively, her partner may press from one side while you meet that pressure from the other side. If she is sidelying, then press the ilium medially toward the bed with your forearm.

♦ ♦ ♦ ♦

Throughout the ages and in most cultures, women have pushed from a squatting or supported squatting position. As birth became more medicalized this century, the recumbent (lithotomy) position became popular with doctors. Modern Western women are rediscovering the squatting and semirecumbent positions. Squatting has been shown to widen the pelvic outlet by up to 28%. Squatting women have shorter labors, with less pain, less need for labor stimulants such as pitocin, fewer and less severe perineal tears, and fewer episiotomies.[46] Because a full squat will not be comfortable for some women, provide equipment or support for a modified squat if desired. A low stool, the side rail of a bed, pillows behind her knees, or partners and other family members often provide the support to accomplish an effective modified squat position.

When birth is imminent, labor attendants will need to have unobstructed access to the laboring woman. When the baby's head begins to first appear, the midwife or physician may apply moist, warm compresses and perineal massage to aid in readying the perineal tissues for maximum stretch with minimum damage. If the birth attendant will support the perineum with her fingers, this helps to alleviate the pressure and allows more time for the tissues to stretch without tearing, and may eliminate the need for an episiotomy. Visualizations and relaxation of the pelvic floor and adductors may encourage opening and reduce the burning pain of the baby "crowning," as the head is born. Since the head is the largest part, most risk of perineal damage passes once the head is out, although occasionally the shoulders will cause a tear. Breech babies are problematic not only for perineal integrity, but also for other safety factors for both the mother and the baby.

An episiotomy is justified when a rapid birth or delivery by forceps is needed, as when the baby's head is too large for the mother, or a tear near or in the urethra seems imminent. In 1995 episiotomy was the most frequently performed surgical procedure in the US. Canadian rates appear to be significantly lower, at 37.7% of all women.[47] Despite the fact that the official position of ACOG is that the routine use of episiotomy is no longer recommended as a standard practice, as many as 90% of first time mothers having hospital births will have an episiotomy. Home births or those at birthing centers under midwifery care have an estimated episiotomy rate of about 10% to 15%.[48] Once she is in labor, you can best help her to maintain an intact perineum by reducing her need for medications, assisting her in finding an instinctively effective pushing position, and maximizing relaxation of her legs and pelvic floor. Assist in reducing muscle tension in her face, neck, and shoulders as she tenses to push. Offer encouraging words or quiet support as she experiences the miraculous intensity of her baby's birth.

"One of my clients and her husband were very anxious that the birth of their first child should be gentle and with as little medical intervention as possible. The labor was very intense, and first stage went very quickly. I used every massage technique I knew to keep the muscles of her hip girdle relaxed. At one point in second stage fetal heart tones diminished several times with very slow recovery after contractions. I immediately had the mother take a chest-to-knees position with her head totally down, and the baby's heart tone returned to normal. During the next contraction we kept the mother in this position. I instructed her to arch her back like a cat while she pushed only as much as she felt was necessary. The father reassured her and patterned breathing for her while I pressed her upper iliac crests together as hard as I could. The doctor was delighted with the results.

We continued this procedure through two more contractions. Then she shifted to her left side with her right leg supported for birth of the baby's head and finally she curled on her back for the shoulders and body of a beautiful, healthy boy. Both baby and mother were very tired. The parents are grateful that it did not end in a cesarean and feel that we all worked well together as a team for the best possible outcome of this birth." — Carroll Patterson, registered massage therapist and doula, Austin, TX

THIRD STAGE LABOR

Within five to ten minutes the strongest uterine contractions of the entire labor shrink the uterus enough to detach the now obsolete placenta and expel it. These afterpains are often very painful, or they may be unnoticeable as the mother joyously focuses on and cuddles her newborn. At this point many women also feel gratefully relieved and disoriented, and she may even begin to tremble involuntarily. Help her to breathe deeply, and remain with her if needed. You may wish to recede into the background for the first minutes to an hour after the birth then proceed with postpartum massage or leave. (See Chapter 5.) This will maximize the new family's bonding with each other, as will encouraging them to have as much "cuddle time" as they'd like in their first weeks together.

CESAREAN BIRTH

Since 1970, U.S. rates of birth by abdominal surgery, or cesarean section, have risen from 5.5 % to over 20% in 1995, and even higher in more affluent areas. These rates are down from their peak of 24.7% in 1988; Canadian rates are similar.[49] Physicians usually perform cesarean sections for the following reasons: failure of labor to progress; pelvic/cephalic disproportion; breech presentations; fetal distress; maternal illnesses, such as diabetes; maternal communicable diseases, such as herpes; medical emergencies, such as prolapsed umbilical cord; doctor or maternal preference; and previous cesarean births (although vaginal birth after previous cesarean, or VBAC, is possible in many cases, and its frequency has risen to 35.5%.) Somatic practitioners are likely to have the opportunity to support a cesarean birth, but their role may be quite different.

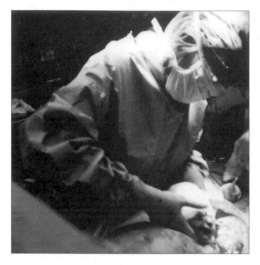

With a planned cesarean, the mother may or may not go into labor spontaneously. If she does labor before surgery, assist as in a vaginal birth by providing nurturing, facilitative touch, emotional comfort, and relaxation and pain management techniques mentioned above. After a prolonged or difficult labor, a woman and her partner are usually devastated if an unplanned, emergency cesarean is necessary. A deep sense of failure, guilt, sorrow, and anger is a counterpoint to their profound relief and joy when a healthy baby and mom are the result.

As she is being prepared for surgery, help her to relax, to move toward resolution of any negativity she feels about the procedure, and to focus on the most positive outcome for her and her baby. Whether planned or unplanned, you generally will not accompany her into the operating room as usually only one person is allowed, and most women prefer their partner's support. Turn your attention to other family members, or rejuvenate yourself for the immediate postpartum work that she may desire.

If needed in the operating room, you probably will only be able to make contact with one of her hands, and her head and neck. The other will be attached to IV's and various monitors, and both arms will be restrained. The attending anesthesiologist usually occupies most of the area at her head as she lies on her back on the operating table. Help her to breathe as deeply as possible, and remind yourself to do likewise, to reduce stress. Eye contact and gentle, yet firm hand holding or stroking are usually possible. This will communicate caring, soothing attention to her as she eagerly awaits her baby's birth. With her abdomen concealed from your view, incisions are made in the abdomen and uterus. Ask for the drape to be lowered if she wants to see her baby as he is born. Help her to snuggle him for a few minutes if possible as the incision is closed.

SELF-CARE FOR LABOR ASSISTANTS

*P*ractitioners assisting at labors must adapt easily and quickly to ever-changing concerns, needs, and even crises. Once-effective techniques may become useless as a labor progresses. An extended first stage labor requiring every "trick in the book" to keep it progressing may be followed by a rapid second stage that demands fast action from the entire birthing group. One contraction may require soft, gentle facial strokes, and for the next you must lean your entire body weight against a painful sacrum.

Since needs and desires for touch vary greatly during labor, it is not uncommon for the laboring woman to reject massage during part or all of the labor. Take such opportunities to rest and refresh yourself. Or allow yourself to be the relaxation expert for the entire birthing group, including family and other professionals. Relaxing or rejuvenating an exhausted father or an overworked midwife can greatly facilitate the labor.

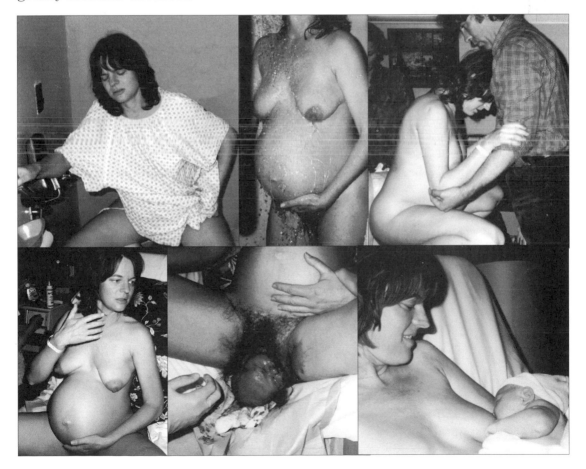

You may find that some medical personnel, family members, or friends do not welcome you. You may need to tactfully and respectfully influence their behaviors when, though well-meaning, they become intrusive or distracting to the woman's experience. Occasionally situations develop where, by default, lack of trust in their ability, or your own control issues, you begin to assume these individuals' roles. Careful, respectful, and appropriate communications are necessary to negotiate the most responsible resolution of these situations. You will want to function so that couple and family relationships are supported and enhanced by your unique contribution to the birth.

Since labors may last from two to 42 hours or more, the somatic practitioner must have great endurance. Remember to eat, stay hydrated, and take mini-breaks for stretching and tension relief when possible. Efficient body mechanics help to conserve energy and reduce overuse injuries, especially to the hands, wrists, and back. Reduce strain to your back from leaning over low, wide hospital beds by adjusting the bed height and having her close to the bedsides when possible. A rolling stool can be very handy, too. When using deep, sustained pressure, as for back labor, align hand, wrist and shoulder joints. Use elbows, knuckles, knees, and legs whenever possible. For long labors, teach others who are willing to perform techniques so that you may rest. Prior to labor, teaching partners labor massage techniques according to their ability and knowledge level is highly recommended.

Labor Massage Techniques to Teach Partners
Abdominal effleurage
Specific foot reflexes
Counterpressure to sacrum
Pelvic press
Reflexive toe squeeze
Contraction distraction technique
Kneading the shoulders and neck

Be prepared for the slim, but real possibility that you may be the only person present when the baby is born. If her partner and medical personnel are not available, call 911 if birth seems imminent at her home, and enlist other motorists to do so if in a car. Reassure the mother, and remain calm. If this is a rapid birth, encourage her not to push, and have her lie on her side. Prepare to safely catch the baby, wipe his face, and keep him warm. If he does not breathe spontaneously within seconds, wipe him again, rub him briskly, and slap his feet. Be sure to lay him prone with nothing obstructing his nose or mouth. Do not worry about cutting the cord.

A high degree of knowledge about birthing is essential to be an effective massage therapist for laboring women. Take at least one childbirth education class, and read voraciously. Complete a comprehensive perinatal class that includes labor massage therapy demonstrations, practice, and videos. Many practitioners may wish to complete auxiliary training as a childbirth assistant (doula). (See Resources appendix.)

Expect utterly unexpected events and outcomes. Even the most prepared, healthy, positive woman, who appears to have done everything "right," can have a very difficult, complicated labor that progresses very differently than anticipated. If this occurs, you may feel as though you failed her, or even caused some of her difficulties. Frightening events and strange equipment and procedures may disrupt your composure and focus. Your own personal issues regarding birthing or other "emotional baggage" may arise to disrupt your ability to be fully present with your client.

Develop your regrouping and concentration skills to be more prepared for these moments. Establish support for yourself to "debrief" after each labor so that you may unburden yourself of any negative feelings you may have developed. Record the labor in your client's chart as soon as possible after the birth. Reviewing the events of the labor with the mother enhances the assimilation of this multifaceted transformation that you have shared.

> *"This summer I was interrupted by my client three weeks before her due date announcing that she was in labor. (The phone rang on the boat just after I had wiped out water skiing!) Driving to the hospital, disappointed that I was missing my niece's birthday lake party, I'm wondering, is it really worth it? The long hours that can be involved, sometimes through the night, sleeping for a little while in a chair or not sleeping at all. Yet, I never feel more 'on' as a pregnancy massage therapist, whether I'm working points intensely on the sacrum or only relaxation work in between contractions. During the actual birth, the emotions, the awe – I know clearly why I love being a massage therapist and doula. It's a wonderful feeling to be so appreciated by the new parents for my presence at their birth. I leave the hospital exhausted, but very fulfilled."*
> — Sheri Danzig, neuromuscular therapist, doula, Atlanta, GA

MASSAGE THERAPY FOR LABOR

	FIRST STAGE			SECOND STAGE	THIRD STAGE
Early Phase	Active Phase		Transition Phase	Pushing to Birth	Placental Separation and Expulsion
0 cm	3 cm		7 cm	10 cm	

Facilitate General Relaxation

Visualization & imagery	Foot reflexology		"Grounding"	Reduce lactic acid buildup	Abdominal breathing
Abdominal breathing	Face & hand massage		Eye contact		
Craniosacral techniques			Reassurance		
Swedish/Esalen massage					

Relieve Localized Painful Areas

Pressure and pleasurable techniques to tight areas

Sensate focusing

Abdominal effleurage

Open mouth exhale with jaw massage and vocalizations

Focus on spinal and pelvic areas

Contraction distraction

"Back labor" techniques

Acupressure toe points

Rhythmic movement

Focus on adductors, pelvic floor, cramp relief in arms and legs

Perineal massage

Sounding

Stimulate Progress of Labor

Uterine foot reflexes

Acupressure points

Gravity-assisted positions

Support positioning changes

Rhythmic movement

Toe grasp

Pelvic press

Encourage gravity-assisted positions

Chapter

5

Postpartum Bodywork

With her newborn warmly snuggled against her, a postpartum woman moves into motherhood. While both exhilarated and exhausted, she must grapple with many changes and challenges in the days and months ahead. She must adapt physiologically and structurally to her non-pregnant state. In spite of her own discomfort and emotional state, her baby demands 24-hour care. She must adjust to changes in relationships with her partner, older children, other family members, and friends. If labor and the birth were not as she expected, then disappointment, guilt, and grief may haunt her.

Birthing a baby is one of life's most extraordinary experiences, a significant rite of passage that generates profound meaning, both conscious and unconscious. It is physically, emotionally, and spiritually transforming. A knowledgeable somatic practitioner can enhance a woman's assimilation of these changes. This chapter explains the physiological, emotional, and structural challenges of the immediate and long-term postpartum period. It elaborates safety protocols for therapeutic bodywork and massage, and sidebars detail several essential techniques for effective postpartum sessions. Pursue qualified instruction in all methods prior to using them postnatally. The author's comprehensive certification workshops further develop these and other specific postpartum techniques.

ADJUSTMENTS AND HEALING
Fatigue, wastes, and pain

*W*ithin hours of the emotional rush of meeting her newborn, counting fingers and toes and gently stroking velvety skin, most mothers will feel exhausted. Napping whenever the baby sleeps and extended family time are usually restorative and bonding for all. Work outside the home and cooking, cleaning, and other household activities, must be given low priority, or handled by someone else.

New mothers and their families need reliable, sustained care for many weeks or months to maximize postpartum recovery and foster family development. Unfortunately, extended postpartum assistance is not available to many women in North America. Fragmented families and inadequate social policies often leave mothers and their newborns isolated, with minimal attention to their many postpartum needs. In other cultures, notably Holland, Sweden, India, and Malaysia, family or social support services provide more long-term, restorative assistance to new families.[1, 2]

Rest provides the downtime needed to recuperate from perinatal exertions and physiological changes. Between the second and fifth days postpartum, a woman will double her daily norm of one and a half quarts of urine output. Perspiring heavily in that first postpartum week, she will lose up to five pounds of excess perinatal interstitial fluid. Heavy elimination flushes lactic acid and other metabolic wastes from sore muscles and aids in removing medication residues. Pitocin, or other medications that improve uterine contractablity, cause edema for several days. Episodes of shakiness and involuntary vibration, such as occur immediately after birth, are common for several days to several weeks.

Labor can be likened to playing a game of football on both the offensive and defensive teams. Many mothers feel the exhaustion, musculoskeletal strain, and pain of an athlete, depending on their labor's length and difficulty. Women whose labors were induced and those who did much commanded pushing often feel most battered afterwards. Awkward, sustained labor positions often result in mild to severe pain. A woman's pelvic size, shape, and its relationship to her baby's head size and position affects the degree of pelvic ligament strain incurred during labor. The sacroiliac, sacrotuberous, and coccxygeal ligaments and the symphysis pubis are especially vulnerable as the baby is pressed down the birth canal. Injury to these soft tissues often contributes to immediate and/or recurring periods of back pain. Occasionally cephalopelvic disproportion results in a dislocated or broken coccyx.

While many women have no negative postpartum responses to epidural anesthesia, others experience headache and backache. They are more prone to headaches, including migraine, than women who labored without these types of regional anesthetics. Some may suffer a severe headache that lasts for several days to weeks after a spinal block or an epidural. These spinal headaches are probably caused by minute cerebral spinal fluid leaks at the injection site.

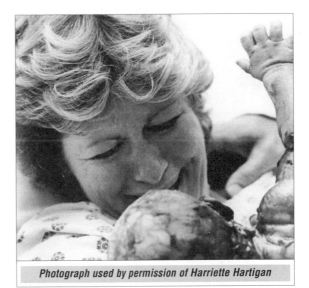

Photograph used by permission of Harriette Hartigan

Epidurals also are associated with postpartum backache, both temporary and long-term.[3] The anesthesia itself may cause achiness, stiffness, and tactile sensitivity. The insertion site is frequently tender, eliciting a psychological protectiveness of this area of her back. Immobility and positioning during administration, injury to the spinal cord membranes, or sustained, strained positions when her pelvis and legs are numb may also have created lumbar, sacral, or pelvic pain.[4] Occasionally some anesthesia accidentally enters the spinal fluid rather than the epidural space, and numbness or tingling may occur for several weeks, or longer.

Within minutes of her baby's birth, powerful uterine contractions expel the placenta and end labor. Immediate, deep, and often painful massage of the uterus by a birth attendant ensures muscular constriction of the vessels of the placental site to prevent hemorrhaging. For many weeks the postpartum uterus will continue to shrink through uterine muscle contractions (involution). These afterpains help her uterus adjust to a non-pregnant state. They continue vasoconstriction in the uterus, expel any remaining clots and dissolved uterine muscle tissue, and complete involution of the uterus almost to its former, plum-like size.

These afterpains may be so intense that they require focused attention to relaxation and abdominal breathing, especially if she is breastfeeding. Because prolactin, the hormone that stimulates milk production, also activates uterine contractions, breastfeeding women are less prone to postpartum hemorrhage. If synthetic oxytocin is necessary for sufficient uterine involution, contractions are often more painful. They also are more painful after second and subsequent births.[5] Postpartum afterpains produce a vaginal discharge of blood and tissue (lochia). Initially bright red, the color of this essentially neutral-smelling lochia will become brown, then more pale, finally ending in three to six weeks after the birth.

With a vaginal birth most women experience some tenderness, bruising, and at least superficial microtears of the vaginal mucosa, humorously known as "skid marks." In addition to these brushburns, some suffer actual tears of the skin, connective tissue, and pelvic floor muscles. Anywhere from one stitch to, in rare cases, several dozen stitches may have been necessary. If she had an episiotomy, her stitched perineum is usually sore and itchy. This tenderness will dissipate over several weeks, as long as the episiotomy or tear suturing was well executed. When she sneezes, coughs, or laughs she may leak some urine until she tones the stretched pelvic floor muscles.

Extended bearing down in second stage labor may have created or exacerbated rectal hemorrhoids. Irregular eating, fluid level imbalances, hormonal adjustments, perineal pain, and fear of pain usually combine to impede bowel movements in the first postpartum days, making constipation common.

The health benefits of breastfeeding for mother, baby, and society are very compelling. Breastfeeding reduces infant mortality and morbidity, improves children's IQs and protects against several diseases. Mothers who breastfeed have a reduced risk of breast cancer, less osteoporosis, and less absenteeism at work because their babies are healthier.[6] These benefits have led the American Academy of Pediatrics to recently recommend that "breastfeeding continue for at least 12 months, and thereafter for as long as mutually desired."[7] Despite these benefits, some women will need to or prefer to bottlefeed because of health concerns, conflicts with work or their partner, or other personal reasons.

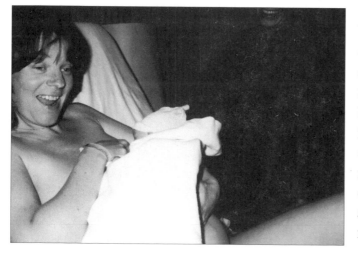

If she chooses to nurse her baby, he is usually able and eager to do so immediately after being born. In fact, Swedish research showed that babies are capable, by the inborn step and rooting reflexes, of reaching the breast and nursing unassisted. When left on their mothers' abdomens after an unmedicated birth, most are able to crawl across their mother's abdomens, locate her nipple, and self-attach to feed.[8] If medications and/or separation were necessary, most babies will successfully breastfeed with mother's help. Some medically stable preemies may even breastfeed, warmed by skin to skin contact with the mother, (Kangaroo Kare) and go home sooner after birth.[9]

Feeding her newborn is often one of a mother's greatest pleasures; however, if a mother breastfeeds, changes in her breasts may initially create discomfort. As the baby sucks, her nipples can become sore, blistered, or cracked, particularly if he does not get a good latch on the breast.

Perinatally, the breasts secrete a highly nutritive, immunologically-rich substance called colostrum. By 72 hours after birth, her breasts begin to swell and produce milk. This breast engorgement continues until the baby's demand for milk regulates the supply, though she may still become engorged after long intervals between feedings. Warm shower water, heat, and massage can ease

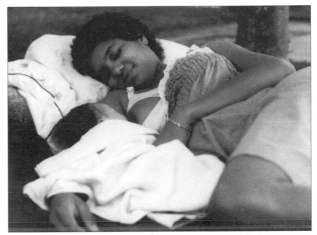

engorgement, help prevent blockage of milk ducts, and help avoid breast infections (mastitis). Babies whose mothers receive labor analgesia, including epidurals, have more breastfeeding difficulties than babies of unmedicated births.[10] If breastfeeding is problematic because she worries over milk supply, struggles with relaxing enough for let-down of the milk from the glands to the nipple, or has other nursing difficulties, she may want to seek advice from a lactation consultant or her local La Leche League (see Resources appendix).

When women prefer bottlefeeding, are unable to breastfeed, or a sudden change to bottlefeeding becomes necessary, medications are available which terminate milk production and reduce breast engorgement. During these 14 days of medication, she is at increased risk for blood clot formation if hormonal inhibitors are used. Other medications can decrease blood pressure and cause nausea, headaches, and dizziness.[11] Some women may prefer non-pharmacological alternatives to stop milk production, such as ice packs to the breasts and a tight binder or bra.

Postpartum Pain and Complaints	
Exhaustion	Musculoskeletal pain and headaches
Uterine involution, afterpains, and lochia	Perineal pain, "skid marks", or stitches
Breastfeeding discomforts	Hemorrhoids, constipation, and other digestive system discomforts

Cesarean birth

*T*he 20% of American women who birth by cesarean section have additional postpartum concerns since they are also recovering from major abdominal surgery.[12] The abdomen and tissue surrounding the incision are initially swollen, and may be either numb or painful. Uterine involution hurts more following cesarean birth, because pitocin usually is necessary to stimulate adequate contractions. Air trapped under the diaphragm during the surgery may create sharp discomfort under the scapula. Abdominal pain from intestinal gas is often excruciating. As detailed previously, spinal anesthesia can cause postoperative difficulties and pain.

Practically every movement made after a cesarean birth is painful: standing, walking, lifting, and holding the baby. It is, however, gentle, frequent movement that produces the most pain relief and improves circulation. She may start by wiggling her feet and sliding her legs in bed. Brief walks, within six to 12 hours after surgery promote peristalsis, hasten the incision healing, improve bladder tone, and reduce the chance of postsurgical complications such as thrombophlebitis and pneumonia.[13]

Because ordinary activities are more difficult after a cesarean, a high bed, crib, and changing table are essential to reduce abdominal muscle strain. Even with this furniture above waist height, others initially may need to care for the newborn. Hot packs over the incision and a lap pillow during feedings will help to heal and protect the incision. Even more than the vaginal birth mother, she needs many naps, extensive assistance with daily tasks, and nurturing, attentive care.

Cesarean Birth Concerns
Pain from incision, involution, and abdominal and intestinal gas
Extreme fatigue, low energy
Need for movement, gentle exercise, and other comfort measures
Emotional recovery / loss of control
Increased risk of thrombophlebitis and pneumonia

Many post-cesarean mothers feel very disappointed about their birth experience. In *The Cesarean Experience*, Kehoe lists the following feelings as more intense after cesarean than after vaginal birth: fear, worry, and anxiety; powerlessness and loss of control; disappointment, shock, and trauma; sense of mutilation or disfigurement; decreased self-esteem; crying, sadness, depression, and defeat; anger, resentment, and blaming others; fatigue; and abandonment.[14] Emotional intensity is escalated if the cesarean was an emergency rather than a planned operation because of fear and an overwhelming sense of loss of control concomitant with unplanned cesareans.[15]

Emotional adjustments and challenges

*W*hether the birth was vaginal or surgical, delightful or traumatic, gratifying or just ordinary, all women undergo postpartum emotional adjustments. Birth is usually elating, despite the many difficulties and possible disappointments that can occur. This elation lasts for hours, sometimes days, after birth while a new mother is exquisitely alert to her newborn, learning his signals, and falling in love. However, most also experience a "come-down" effect after labor's excitement and intensity.

Hormonal changes alone can account for increased mood swings and emotional intensity (lability). Estrogen and progesterone production decrease by 90% within the first three postpartum hours; oxytocin and prolactin levels increase, especially if a woman is breastfeeding. Adjusting to these hormonal changes, plus a drop in blood sugar and tidal volume in the lungs, also increases exhaustion.

A new baby alters every aspect of daily life: eating, sleep cycles, entertainment, work schedules, and homemaking, to name a few. While these changes and new responsibilities are joyous and love-filled, most women have periods of anxiety, dislike, and other negative feelings. Fifty percent to eighty percent of postpartum woman experience the "baby blues," especially in the third to fifth days after the birth.

Common Negative Feelings in the Postpartum Period:			
fear	worry	anxiety	powerlessness
loss of control	disappointment	decreased self-esteem	shock
trauma	depression	defeat	anger
resentment	blaming	sadness	abandonment

The most common postpartum complication, mental illness, occurs in about 5%-15% of Western mothers.[16] Psychologists divide these postpartum mood disorders into four categories with related, yet differing symptoms: postpartum depression, postpartum psychosis, postpartum panic disorder, and postpartum obsessive-compulsive disorder. Sleep disturbances, other than those created by the infant's needs, radical emotional changes, altered eating habits, reduced energy level, an inability to think clearly, and real or fantasized abusive actions are indicative of more than the normal adjustments to life with a new baby.[17]

Physicians consider postpartum mental illnesses to result from hormonal influences on neurotransmitter uptake in the brain's nerve synapses. This imbalance in brain chemistry makes a woman more susceptible to the difficult effects of psychological stresses, lack of support from family or friends, or unrealistic expectations of birth and postpartum life with her baby. She is especially vulnerable if she has a history of chronic or recurring depression.[18] Depressed mothers tend to gaze at, play with, and attend to their infants less frequently than nondepressed mothers do. Recent research has indicated that when depressed mothers massaged their infants, the effects of this neglect were minimized.[19]

Postpartum Emotional Adjustments	
Assimilating the birthing experience	Grief and unexpected outcomes
Demands of infant care	Self-identity
"Baby blues"	Relationship issues with partners, older children, and others
Postpartum mental illnesses	Sexual activity

Since many pregnancies progress and finish differently than the parents anticipate, most women experience at least some disappointment.[20] These unexpected outcomes can range from less serious concerns, such as the labor being over too quickly or missing use of planned equipment or techniques, to greater disappointments like the baby's sex, the use of drugs, or other undesired labor interventions such as cesarean sections. Serious crises can include prematurity, maternal and fetal health crises, genetic defects, perinatal injuries, stillbirths, miscarriages, and neonatal deaths.

A mother whose infant needs intensive care anguishes over her fragile newborn fighting for his life. She may feel shocked, guilty, and torn between bonding with him and distancing herself, hoping to minimize her pain if he dies. Hopes for his survival and worries whether he will be normal turn what was anticipated as a joyful time into an ordeal. She may struggle relentlessly to protect and save him, often ignoring her own postpartum care. Those women who cope best with a newborn in ICU seem to be those who can express their emotions, accept others' help, seek information, and begin an early relationship with the baby (see support agencies, Resources appendix).

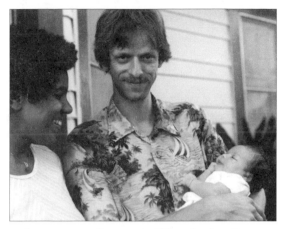

A new mother's relationships with all family members and friends are usually in flux. While she may need additional attention, she may also yearn for solitude and recuperative rest. The desire for more time with her older children and for rest and bonding time with the baby create conflict. She and her partner may have reduced opportunities and perhaps less inclination for intimacy. Her sexual appetite is often drastically different post-partum. Sexual activity before six or more weeks postpartum may be impossible, painful, or anxiety provoking. Women who are in abusive relationships may find that the baby is now also in danger (see referral agencies, Resources appendix). Some women with histories of sexual abuse feel retraumatized by childbirth.[20]

Abdominal and structural changes

With her baby's birth, a woman loses approximately 11 pounds: eight pounds of baby, one or two pounds of placenta, and another two pounds of amniotic fluid and blood. Excess fluid excretion through increased urination and perspiration lightens her by another five pounds in the first postpartum week. As the uterus involutes, it shrinks from 2.3 pounds at term to three ounces by the sixth week postpartum, for a total initial weight loss of 15-18 pounds.

While these changes reduce much of the anterior weight load, she gains a few pounds of breast tissue and milk. Breastfeeding, however, will gradually account for further weight loss as milk production depletes fat stores in her thighs, buttocks, and abdomen. Regular, appropriate exercise and proper nutrition are fundamental to a mother's return to her pre-pregnant size.

The postpartum abdomen feels doughy, flaccid, and is often pendulous. The skin and connective tissue are stretched, loose, and often etched with stretch-marks. Hypotoned, stretched abdominal muscles are peppered with trigger points and weakened by rectus abdominus separation. Displacement of the intestines, bladder, and other abdominal organs may persist.

A postpartum woman may feel some disorientation, lack of balance, and continuing back pain. With her proprioceptors set to pregnancy's anterior weight load, she often retains her pregnant posture. She still tilts her chin and hyperextends her neck, which creates tension in the cervical extensors. Her pectoral girdle continues its anterior collapse, and her upper rib cage leans back while her lumbar spine curves excessively. With these misalignments and referred pain from both anterior and posterior trigger points, she may continue to experience back and pelvic pain, especially in the sacroiliac and lumbosacral areas. She may still waddle rather than fluidly flex and extend at the hip when she walks due to excessive external hip rotation and disuse or spasm of the iliopsoas.

Unrelenting childcare activities exacerbate any postural deviations and soft tissue disorganization. If she is breastfeeding, she may spend 40 hours a week in that activity alone. Most women suffering prenatal carpal tunnel syndrome will experience relief perinatally; however, older mothers of two or more children tend to develop wrist pain while breastfeeding.[23] Diapering, consoling, carrying, and interacting with her baby are equally as demanding. She can reduce musculoskeletal strain by obtaining assistance in these tasks and by observing proper body mechanics, especially immediately after the birth.

GUIDELINES AND PRECAUTIONS FOR PRACTITIONERS

While most women can benefit from massage therapy immediately after birth, they usually are eager to bond with their newborn, to begin reconfiguring their family, and to rest. Begin postpartum massage therapy as soon as desired after birth, if no complications have occurred. New mothers appreciate attention to both emotional and physical concerns. Provide an open, empathetic environment, and emphasize relaxation massage, rich in abdominal and pain relieving strokes.

Both practitioner and mother are more responsive to maternal needs when someone else cares for the baby. Though many newborns sleep throughout a session, the squirming, grunting, and other infant behaviors are inevitably distracting. With the baby securely in another's care, mom more effectively lets go of all but her own concerns, and the practitioner can focus on attending to her. If the baby must accompany her, he may be on the table too. With a fussy infant, sometimes chair work and body mechanics guidance must replace tablework, or infant massage, not mother massage, is needed. Be flexible to create a productive session.

Equipment and positioning modifications are usually necessary with postpartum women. Tenderness and leakage of milk require additional breast supports and towels to protect the head end of the massage table. Most women prefer to keep their bra on. Augment prone positioning with additional chest and/or abdominal pillows, or use a Contoured bodyCushion® with larger breast recesses. Sidelying positioning is often the most comfortable for posterior work. Provide additional pillow support under a sidelying, post-cesarean client's abdomen to prevent uncomfortable tugging on the incision. Avoid supine position until any tenderness around the epidural site has dissipated.

Postpartum Positioning	
Supine:	Knee bolsters
Sidelying:	Firm pillows or Contoured bodyCushion® to maintain horizontal alignment
Prone:	Reduce pressure on breasts; after cesarean birth release
Comfort Factors:	Breast or incision tenderness
	Milk leakage
	Epidural site
	Baby

Continue to observe all pregnancy contraindications concerning circulatory massage therapy methods, especially on the legs and pelvis. Blood clot risks remain high until eight to ten weeks postpartum as the fibrolynic activity level favors closure of the placental site to prevent hemorrhaging.[24] While many types of abdominal massage are beneficial, carefully avoid pressure in the inguinal area, especially in the first week, as clots are common in the femoral and iliac veins. Be especially cautious when symptoms of thrombophlebitis occur, such as leg, chest, or lower abdomen pain, or heat or swelling in the legs. Remember that many leg thrombi are asymptomatic.

When maternal complications requiring restricted activity and additional bed rest have occurred, risks of pneumonia and thrombi escalate dramatically. Post-cesarean women have a two to three times higher risk of thromboembolism than those who birthed vaginally. Postpartum operative procedures such as tubal ligation also tend to foster elevated clot development.[25] Eliminate all leg massage until her healthcare provider has released her from maternity care. Delay most abdominal techniques for post-cesarean women, unless working directly under medical supervision, until her incision is healed, and she receives a release.

In addition to these post-cesarean and thrombi complications, other postpartum complications include hemorrhaging; uterine, breast, incision, kidney, or other infections; and mental illness. Warning signs of these complications are usually identifiable. Uterine infections will result in fever and a peculiar color or odor to lochia. If the lochia becomes bright red and abdominal pain, beyond tenderness, occurs, hemorrhaging is suspected. Refer any woman who reports bright red blood (except for immediately postpartum or immediately after extended periods of lying down) or any foul smell to the lochia to her physician or midwife.

An unusual increase in urinary frequency or burning during urination may signal a bladder or kidney infection. Breast infections usually result in tender, inflamed lumps in the breast and flu-like symptoms, including chills or fever. While reflexive work may promote healing in these areas, refer her for medical treatment for these symptoms before performing massage therapy.

Be alert to any indication of severe emotional distress. Warning signs of postpartum mental illness include: difficulty in getting out of bed; rapid weight gain or loss; sustained use of alcohol, sedatives, or other medications; serious accidents related to fatigue or inattention; planning or attempting injury to herself or others; uncontrollable crying and mood shifts.[26] Refer women with any symptoms of postpartum complications to their physician or midwife and ask them to provide written release for massage therapy.

Summary of Contraindications to Postpartum Massage Therapy

Modify leg and abdominal massage to prevent dislodging clots.

No leg massage if birthing complications require bed rest.

With cesarean births, no abdominal techniques until incision heals and with a medical release.

No massage without physician's release when maternal complications have occurred.

POSTPARTUM MASSAGE THERAPY
Nurturing and emotional support

*P*rovide a special time to focus on "mothering the mother" by creating a calming ambiance and listening with your hands and your heart. Many somatic practices promote postpartum relaxation, including Swedish and Esalen circulatory styles, connective tissue massage (*Bindegewebsmassage*), foot zone therapy, and passive movements performed rhythmically, with fluidity and focus.

Many women enjoy a technique modified from the practices of Mexican midwives which they accomplish by systematically wrapping their *robozo* (shawl) around the new mother.[27] Somatic practitioners may simulate the "closing" effect of this practice by applying firm, sustained, medial directed pressure bilaterally, working from head to toe, as though pressing her back together. Other women may appreciate the extra support of an abdominal binder or a light girdle until postpartum healing is more complete.

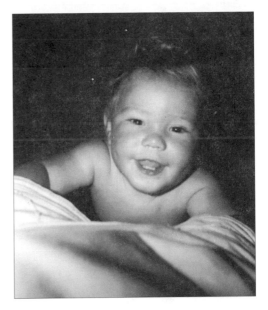

Responsive, soothing touch that communicates nurturing enhances her pleasure in being a mother and often prompts the unburdening of any negative feelings about the birth and postpartum life. Listening with a nonjudgmental, supportive attitude can provide just the atmosphere for her to tell her story honestly, including her disappointments, angers, fears, and regrets.

Assist grieving women as they navigate through the typical stages of grief recovery: denial, sadness, anger, and reconciliation. Sheila Kitzinger sensitively describes the many possible sources of postpartum grief: loss of the pregnancy experience and the special anticipation of gestation; disappointment when birthing and parenting expectations are unmet; loss of the "dream baby" as she adjusts to the real baby; reduced romance and intimacy with her partner; loss of self-identity or of her own childhood, particularly poignant if she was neglected or abused; and loss of her former lifestyle.[28]

Remember that not all postpartum mothers have live babies. Some chose to terminate their pregnancies through abortion, and approximately 20% of all known pregnancies end in miscarriage; 1% of babies are stillborn; and another 1% die within hours or days of birth.[29] Sudden infant death syndrome (SIDS or "crib death") inexplicably kills another 1% of babies less than one year old. The grieving mothers of these infants are still in postpartum recovery, regardless of how or when their loss occurred.

Postpartum massage therapy techniques assist her in adjusting physiologically and emotionally. Because she has experienced the death of her baby, her feelings range the spectrum in intensity and texture. Avoid minimizing her grief with well-intended, but insensitive, comments such as: "It was meant to be" or "You can always have another." A heartfelt "I'm so sorry" is more appreciated. Offer her compassionate, caring attention without prying, and focus on the same types of physiological recovery as those mothers with live infants. (See active listening and somatoemotional integration techniques, Chapter 3, and support agencies in Resources appendix.)

Physiological and musculoskeletal adjustment

> *"Rhonda began having spasms in the SI and sacral areas that "took her breath away" during the last two months of her pregnancy and continued postpartum. She called when Mackenna was five weeks old seeking relief and infant massage instruction. At this point she was afraid to go upstairs in her own home, needed help with outside errands, and feared dropping the baby when the pain hit. After her first infant massage lesson, I sculpted the tensor fascia lata and all of the other hip muscles, focusing on piriformis, iliotibial tract, and quadratus lumborum, followed by deep fanning to these areas. The immediate relief she experienced lasted for three days, then intermittent twinges returned. Our second session was similar, with additional deep work in her upper back and pelvis. She's been pain-free for six weeks now, and her confidence and mobility are normal."* — Linda Hickey, registered massage therapist, Calgary, Alberta, Canada

*F*ull body sessions of Swedish and lymphatic drainage facilitate restoration of normal physiology by opening capillary beds and increasing cellular respiration, cleansing residual metabolic wastes from labor's exertions and any residual anesthesia, and pumping excess fluids from interstitial spaces into general circulation for elimination. Connective tissue massage, zone therapy, and other reflexive modalities also stimulate the body's return to normal functioning.

Remind her to exercise the pelvic floor with Kegel exercises immediately postpartum to promote healing, aid in the recovery of sphincter control, and to prevent uterine prolapse. Many women find a warm water sitz bath temporarily soothing, while cold packs usually offer more extended relief from perineal pain.[30]

If her breasts engorge, she may use cold packs or towels wrapped around each breast to reduce swelling. While breast massage therapy is generally considered outside of practitioners' scope of practice or illegal in some areas of the U.S., clients may wish to learn breast self-massage.[31, 32] Teach her to first perform several minutes of circular fingertip kneading in the lymphatic areas of her axilla. She may then continue with three rounds of fingertip circles around each breast as if performing a self-examination for unusual lumps. Finally, teach her to take the entire breast between her hands for gentle kneading. Massaging her breasts may create the comfort and experience she needs to learn to manually express her milk when needed.

♦ ♦ FOOT REFLEXOLOGY ♦ ♦

Reflex massage to specific foot zones may facilitate postpartum relaxation and recovery. Include zone therapy in each postpartum session, and teach her to work with specific zones daily, perhaps as she breastfeeds.

1. Use the side of the thumb and/or a finger to create bone-on-bone pressure into the foot. Travel with tiny, overlapping movements, compressing the skin and nerves of the foot against the bones. Imagine that your finger moves like a tiny inchworm as you cover each area three times.

2. Work on the entire foot, focusing on the following postpartum complaint areas: neck, upper back, spine, pelvis and sacrum, colon, bladder, uterus, and breasts.

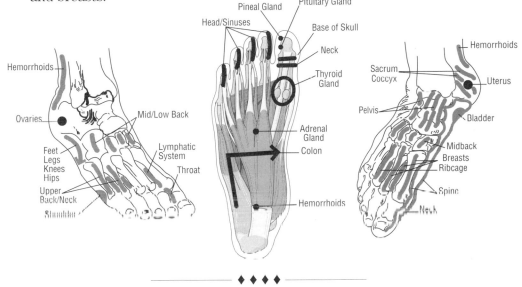

♦ ♦ ♦ ♦

Twice daily applications of vitamin E oil in the first three postpartum months is recommended for stretchmarks.[33] Connective tissue massage and skin rolling may also be helpful in normalizing the abdominal skin and connective tissue. Use gentle tapotement on the abdominal muscles to stimulate tone in these slack muscles. Tapping and hacking will activate proprioceptors, creating some reflexive tightening of the rectus, oblique, and transverse abdominals. The neurological stimulation combined with appropriate exercise will help reduce the jelly-like feel of many postpartum bellies.

Deep abdominal kneading improves circulation and relieves congestion in organs cramped and displaced during the pregnancy. Encourage her to continue with the uterine massage taught her by her birth attendants to facilitate involution and to prevent hemorrhaging. Delay other abdominal massage techniques until postoperative release when working with post-cesarean women.

In the perinatal period, the stretched rectus abdominus usually separates at the strained, softened linea alba, and it fails to maintain spinal and pelvic alignment. Be alert to the contribution this dysfunction makes to postural imbalance, musculoskeletal pain, and diminished self-image after pregnancy. If she has a separation, guide her to abdominal strengthening while supporting the diastus, as described by Elizabeth Noble, P.T. By reaching across her torso with each hand to hold the opposite edge of the rectus toward the midline she may begin gentle, progressive abdominal strengthening exercises.[34] When correct exercise is performed regularly up to 50 times a day, healing usually occurs within a few weeks. Teach her to roll onto one side when rising from a reclining position, to avoid jack-knife like movements that further strain this vulnerable area.

◆ ◆ DIASTUS RECTI CHECK ◆ ◆

Most women will have an inch to four inches of soft space at the linea alba immediately postpartum. Evaluate the extent of diastus, and continue to monitor her progress in closing this gap.

1. Stand at pelvic level facing your supine client's head. Place the fingertips of your inside hand at umbilical level, paralleling the rectus fibers.
2. Maintaining a gentle pressure, instruct your client to lift her head and upper torso from the table. Check whether and to what extent your fingers fall into any soft space between the tightening rectus.
3. Note any bulging of abdominal contents that may occur in this space with this movement.
4. Any separation of three or more finger widths indicates a need for special care with abdominal exercise and/or future monitoring.

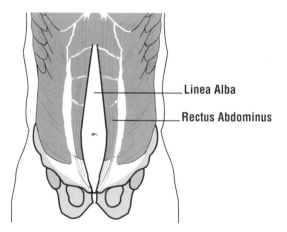

Linea Alba

Rectus Abdominus

◆ ◆ ◆ ◆

♦ ♦ ABDOMINAL TRIGGER POINTS ♦ ♦

During pregnancy the abdominal muscles worked heroically to maintain postural integrity as they stretched over the growing uterus. These muscles are typically replete with trigger points from these strains, especially at and near their attachments. Many of these trigger points refer to organs and to the back, creating abdominal or persistent low and mid-back pain if they are not extinguished.

1. Stand at pelvic level facing the supine client's head. Use several fingertips to create a sawing motion noting any jump response from the client. Especially check locations indicated in the accompanying diagram, including: one to two inches below the xiphoid process; superficial to ribs eight through twelve; inferior to the costal rib cage; medial to

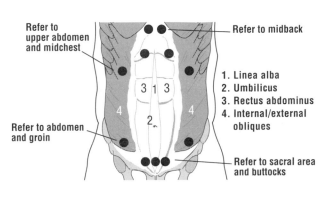

Refer to upper abdomen and midchest

Refer to midback

Refer to abdomen and groin

1. Linea alba
2. Umbilicus
3. Rectus abdominus
4. Internal/external obliques

Refer to sacral area and buttocks

the ASIS; and just superior to the pubic symphysis (with cesarean births, after postpartum release and when scar tenderness diminishes).
2. Confirm that any tender point referring into the abdomen that is not on bone is a muscular trigger point and not organic tenderness. When the client lifts her head and pain increases, that point is a trigger point. If pain decreases, it is organic in nature, so release pressure.
3. Moderate your pressure on an identified trigger point until the pain is no more intense than pleasure on the borderline of pain.
4. Request client feedback of changes in pain intensity. Once her pain dissipates, continue to compress for 7-20 seconds. If possible, stretch the trigger area for 30-60 seconds, or perform localized strokes over the area. Alternately, move client to a position that eliminates the pain, and hold her there for 90 seconds. Slowly return her to her original position.

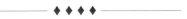

♦ ♦ ♦ ♦

If she had an epidural or spinal, specific attention to the administration site in her upper lumbar spine may be needed in the first month postpartum. Work initially with broad, sweeping, superficial strokes, progressing to deeper, more specific work. Use craniosacral and connective tissue techniques to reduce tenderness and any emotional sensitivity to the area. If she has a spinal headache, use craniosacral techniques on her head, spine, and sacrum. Work head and neck reflexes on the plantar creases of her big toes, and gently reduce tension and trigger points in the head, neck, and back.

Deep tissue sculpting and structural balancing facilitate release of chronic tension in the pelvic and lumbar musculature and shortening of all of the posterior fascial planes. Pay particular attention to the erector spinae, the quadra-

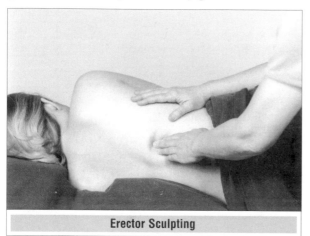

Erector Sculpting

tus lumborum, the lumbodorsal fascia, the piriformis, and other hip movers. These contracted areas also may harbor trigger points. Use neuromuscular therapy, rhythmic and positional movement techniques, and deep tissue methods. (See specific techniques of hip and back sculpting/ trigger points, lumbosacral stretch, and sacroiliac release, Chapter 3.) Guide her standing, seated, and carrying postures to reestablish effortless, graceful alignment and to reduce musculoskeletal strain. Help her to correct the typical anterior tilting pelvis and increased lumbar curvature by strengthening and reeducating her major postural muscles.

Imbalance in the iliopsoas' relationships with the erector spinae and piriformis affects SI joint function and pelvic alignment.[35] The iliopsoas is often not capable of maintaining pelvic alignment throughout the pregnancy. By the postpartum period, it becomes hypertonic and spasmed. Strain to the iliopsoas may have produced myofascial trigger points referring pain into the lower back, and it may need stretching. Alternately, it may be hypotonic if it was incompetent for much of the pregnancy. Some iliopsoas strengthening occurs when the postpartum woman repeatedly reduces the lumbar lordosis by tilting her pelvis posteriorly, using the iliopsoas rather than the gluteal, leg, or upper abdominal muscles. (See pelvic/lumbar alignment, Chapter 3.) As in pregnancy, active and passive pelvic tilts also help relieve lumbar pain.

As both pelvic stabilizer and one of the primary hip flexors, the psoas muscle is integrally involved in gait. Ideally one psoas initiates leg flexion on the pelvis, followed by contraction of the rectus femoris and other quadriceps group muscles. Simultaneously, the contralateral psoas stabilizes the pelvis to avoid excess pelvic rotation and tilting. These two psoas functions become increasingly compromised perinatally. The continuous anterior uterine weight contributes to disuse of the normal psoas functions for walking. Instead, the hip joints begin to externally rotate, and the hip rotators rather than the psoas initiate each step. The resulting "duck walk" or "sailor's roll" is characteristic of both the third trimester and the postpartum period. Use imagery to guide the mother in regaining psoas use and strength and to increase her awareness of this important postural muscle.

♦ ♦ STRUCTURAL BALANCING FOR PSOAS ♦ ♦

Deep tissue sculpting to release myofascial contraction will be especially effective in combination with imagery-guided pelvic tilting. Work in sidelying position, or, if supine, use a large bolster under her knees to relax the abdomen.

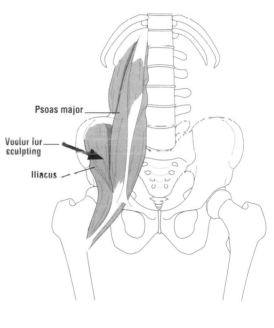

Psoas major

Vector for sculpting

Iliacus

1. Stand at pelvic level facing the client's feet. Use the fingertips of your inside hand to gradually sink into the pelvic bowl just medial to the ASIS. Avoid compressing into the femoral triangle, especially in the first eight to ten postpartum weeks.
2. Continue to carefully compress into abdominals, iliacus, and psoas, creating minimal discomfort. Extinguish any trigger points discovered in each muscle layer.
3. Use imagery to guide her into initiating the pelvic tilt movement, lengthening her lumbar spine, and flexing her hip by activating the iliopsoas against your fingertips.
4. Develop coordination of her movement with her exhalations, and repeat three to ten times.

♦ ♦ ♦ ♦

Many women suffer pregnancy-induced back and neck pain far beyond the postpartum period. Effective massage therapy in the first one to three months after birthing as detailed above may help her to avoid this problem. Women with chronic back pain, who were pregnant years ago, often benefit from similar sessions designed to address these long-standing dysfunctions. The postpartum period is an excellent time to undergo a complete series of structural balancing based on the principles of Ida Rolf or sequential Aston-Patterning® sessions. Encourage her to walk daily and to resume appropriate exercise as soon as possible.

> *"A new client who was 11 days postpartum greeted me at the door bent over and walking like she had been 'in the saddle' for months. I immediately taught her a pelvic tilt without clenching the gluts and abdominals as she had been doing. Hip, ab, and low back deep work were gratefully received, but more than that, the information I had to share was like a lifeline to her. She had been desperately asking every woman she knew 'why do I hurt so much, and why can't I stand straight?' She had enough college anatomy training to understand my descriptions, and, when I isolated the psoas muscle for her, it was like a light going on. She got off my table standing 100% better, but it wasn't just my work. It was the relief that she now understood what was going on, and she had a tool to deal with it."* — Deborah Donaldson, certified massage therapist, Framingham, MA

Post-cesarean birth massage

*T*he woman who has had an operative birth needs special attention to her recovery. In Europe, physicians commonly prescribe lymphatic drainage for their surgical patients to enhance circulation, immunological functioning, and parasympathetic stimulation. With a planned cesarean birth, presurgical work is beneficial, and postsurgical full-body lymphatic drainage techniques can facilitate postoperative recovery.[36]

Encourage deep abdominal breathing. Address pain from gas, constipation, and the incision initially through corresponding zones on her feet. With permission from her healthcare provider, perform connective tissue and other abdominal massage. In initial sessions, thorough yet gentle abdominal kneading helps reestablish peristalsis, ease gas pain, and foster lymphatic flow.[37] Focus techniques on the flexures and on the iliocecal valve areas of the colon. Avoid work that mobilizes the scar until it is completely healed, usually two to three weeks, or until she receives a medical release. Observe other contraindications and precautions for leg and abdominal massage detailed previously.

Use other techniques described in this chapter to nurture, heal, and promote her overall recovery. She may want to inquire about the use of a TENS unit (transcutaneous electrical nerve stimulation) for pain control rather than medications. This physical therapy modality, which operates on the Gate Theory, offers individualized pain management and may decrease intestinal distension and numbness around the incision site.[38]

For incision pain, encourage her to gently place her hands over her clothing and/or the bandages and to create a butterfly-light vibration on the incision. This type of lymphatic drainage technique may begin to reduce surrounding edema, facilitate incision closure, and encourage her to deal with any emotional issues generated by the operation.

Once the staples or stitches are removed and the incision is completely healed, a progression of techniques over several weeks or months can facilitate healing and reduce scar tissue buildup in the various scar layers. With client consent, begin with light, stationary touch and subtle vibration of the skin. Stroke gently with your fingertips from the scar toward the inguinal nodes to drain edemous tissue, and work towards the scar to facilitate tissue repair.[39]

As the client feels physically and emotionally amenable to deeper massage, work progressively with the skin, superficial fascia, deep fascia, and finally the muscle layers. Use fingertip circles to identify areas where the scar is tight, thickened, or immovable, and hold these areas on stretch to prevent and break down adhesions. Progress to a deeper layer only when the more superficial layers of the entire scar are mobile. Numerous sessions will be required before you may friction and roll the scar.

Best results with scars are achieved with work immediately postpartum, although older scars benefit from increased circulation and will become softer. Most importantly, fascial shortening, bunching, and tensions that can produce long-term postural and function imbalances can be reduced.[40]

Preventing pain from childcare activities

*I*nfant care is usually a loved-filled, if sometimes tedious, task. Many aspects of baby care involve innumerable lifting, twisting, and bending movements. These movements are particularly dangerous with muscles and joints still unbalanced by the pregnancy. Many involve extreme forward bending, a movement she has not done for many months. When performed incorrectly, these repetitive actions contribute to lumbar, thoracic, and cervical pain. As the baby grows, its additional weight exacerbates back strain.

As a vital part of preventive care, parents need instruction in proper body mechanics for these activities; teach them prenatally, if possible. Instruct parents to lift their baby as any object should be lifted: protect the spine by bending the knees to reach the infant; lift from the legs by straightening the knees rather than lifting with the back or pectoral girdle; when possible, avoid lifting and twisting the spine simultaneously. Moving the baby in or out of car seats is particularly challenging; instruct them to get into the car if possible before twisting to place or lift their infant.

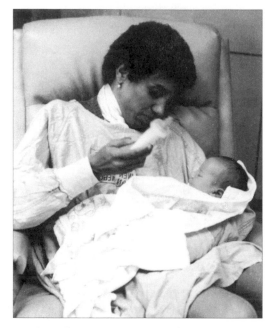

Many parents spend hours each day with their baby cradled in their embracing arms, looking down at their "little miracle." It is mesmerizing to gaze into the soulful eyes and inviting face of a newborn. Unfortunately, this side bending, forward tilting static posture of the neck and head, coupled with the use of the upper back muscles for holding, creates an overuse syndrome, "new parents' neck." Encourage regularly switching from left to right side and periodically lifting and straightening out the neck. When not holding the baby, shoulder rolls, arm stretches, and lifting the back of the head help to relax and stretch these muscles.

Another common neck problem occurs in the night. A new mother dozes off, her neck and upper back crooked, uncovered, and eventually chilled. When she startles awake to a fussy infant after sleeping in this awkward position, the sudden jerking movement wrenches her joints, spasming neck and back muscles.

To reduce strain during feedings, parents should sit with back support in chairs with low arms, if possible, and with sufficient pillows supporting the baby to relax the shoulder. When breastfeeding, the mother should bring the baby to the breast with pillow and armrest support rather than hunching and sidebending her torso.

Breastfeeding mothers will inevitably bring the baby to bed for nocturnal feedings. Encourage her to minimize neck and back strain by sitting up completely, with pillows supporting her lumbar spine, legs, and the baby. She also may lie on her side, again well supported by pillows or her partner at her back. This sidelying position is not only structurally more comfortable for the mother, but is also more conducive to dozing while nursing. She should support the baby on his side using a rolled receiving blanket or wedge. The American Academy of Pediatrics and the SIDS Alliance recommend supine or sidelying sleeping positions for most healthy, full-term infants.[41]

Many parents carry their newborns upright on their upper chest and one shoulder. Frequently the parent then leans posterior, painfully compressing the lumbar spine. In elevating the carrying shoulder, the trapezius and levator scapulae become very tense. Guide parents to drop the carrying shoulder to a more relaxed level and to maintain the spine's vertical alignment. The upper back and shoulder need similar relaxation when using the arm cradle described above.

As the baby gains head and torso control, carrying the baby on the hip is common. While most mothers' hips are wide enough to provide a ledge for the baby to rest, many will shift their weight and pelvis, slinging the carrying hip laterally. This provides additional support for the baby, but it can contribute to back pain from excess strain to the quadratus lumborum, erector spinae, and oblique abdominals. Occasionally, scoliosis of the spine results from this posture.

If the parent cannot hold the infant on one hip while maintaining spinal and pelvic alignment, she may instead carry on the abdomen, facing outward. This carry is easier on the parent's structure, as long as she does not lean posteriorly at the waist. The "football carry", with the baby prone on the forearm, is another alternative. Both of these carries have the additional advantage to the baby of stimulating head and torso strength while providing an alternate view of his world.

Many women discover musculoskeletal relief, increased mobility, and a more content infant by "wearing" their babies in a sling or other cloth carrier. A variety of designs, fabrics, and sizes are available, offering the advantages of Mexican women's *robozos* or other cultures' slings. Resourceful women may create their own inexpensive carrier from old sheets.[42]

In a recent, comprehensive review of all carrier varieties, *Midwifery Today* recommended the front packs Baby Wrap and Baby Bundler to reduce neck and back strain for many women. They also found the Over the Shoulder Baby Holder™ to be a comfortable sling that is easy to use; the NoJo sling to be reliable and widely available; and the Maya wrap notable for its beautiful fabric and flexibility.[42] (See Resources appendix.)

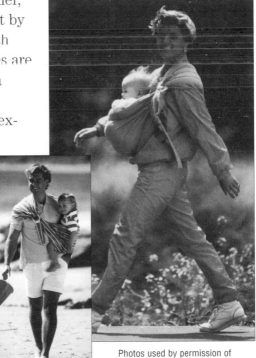

Photos used by permission of
Over the Shoulder Baby Holder™

Advise her to try on carriers until she finds her best fit and to choose a high enough stroller to avoid hunched pushing. Encourage her to avoid dangling a heavy plastic infant seat from one arm. Diapering or lifting the baby from higher changing tables and cribs reduces back strain from bending over. Often the kitchen sink is better for baths than leaning over the bathroom tub.

Massage therapy techniques helpful in reducing childcare strain include: Aston-Patterning®, deep tissue sculpting, passive movement, stretching, and trigger point therapy. Focus on the sternocleidomastoid, the suboccipitals, splenius capitus, levator scapula, supraspinatus, trapezius, rhomboidei, erector spinae group, and quadratus lumborum. Reflexively reduce strained and painful areas by stimulating the related zones of the feet for the back, neck, and shoulders.

> *"Andrea had Connor by cesarean after an unsuccessful, ultra-sound-assisted version to move him out of breech. Her hip that we had worked with at 36 weeks was occasionally painful, but her left pectoral girdle was most problematic from carrying him while attending to other tasks and her three-year-old. Before she undressed, we worked with her standing alignment and alternative ways to carry Connor. In sidelying position, rhythmic passive movements and positional releases began to loosen the shortened and spasmed pectoral girdle structures. Deep tissue sculpting, cross-fiber friction, and lomi-lomi techniques both to the area and to the paravertebral muscles further lengthened fascial planes, reduced fibrous buildup, and increased circulation. She reported the pain completely gone after a very tender trigger point at the rib cage rectus attachment was extinguished. We finished this session on her feet after gentle abdominal work, including a plan to begin progressive scar work at our next session."* — Carole Osborne-Sheets, integrative body therapist, San Diego, CA

Summary of Postpartum Massage Therapy Goals

Nurture and provide emotional support	Restore and normalize abdominal structures
Facilitate restoration of prepregnancy physiology	Facilitate healing from cesarean birth
Alleviate muscle strain/fatigue of labor and birth	Restore normal walking patterns
Promote pelvic floor healing and comfort	Prevent and reduce back and neck pain caused by newborn care
Rebalance pelvic and spinal structural realignment	

CLOSING THOUGHTS

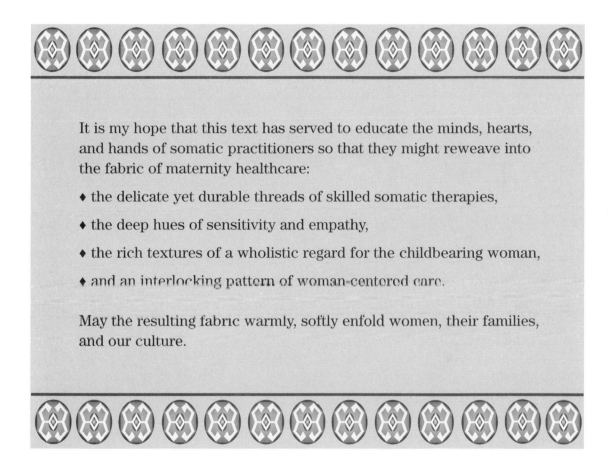

It is my hope that this text has served to educate the minds, hearts, and hands of somatic practitioners so that they might reweave into the fabric of maternity healthcare:

♦ the delicate yet durable threads of skilled somatic therapies,

♦ the deep hues of sensitivity and empathy,

♦ the rich textures of a wholistic regard for the childbearing woman,

♦ and an interlocking pattern of woman-centered care.

May the resulting fabric warmly, softly enfold women, their families, and our culture.

REFERENCES CITED:

Chapter 1, Benefits of Pre- and Perinatal Massage Therapy

1 Helton, A.S., McFarlane, J., & Anderson, E.T. "Battered and pregnant: a prevalence study." *American Journal of Public Health* 77, p. 1337-39.

2 Ventura, S.J. "Trends and variations in first births to older women, 1970-1986." *Vital Health Statisitcs*, 21:1989, p. 47.

3 Harker, Lisa and Thorpe, Karen Ph.D. "The last egg in the basket? elderly primiparity: a review of findings." *Birth*, Vol 19, #1, March, 1992, p. 72.

4 Dick-Read, Grantly, M.D. *Childbirth Without Fear, Fifth Edition*. Harper & Row: NY, 1984, p. 189.

5 Gorsuch, R. and Key, M. "Abnormalities of pregnancy as a function of anxiety and life stress." *Psychosomatic Medicine*, 36:1974, p. 353.

6 Cranden, A. "Maternal anxiety and obstretric complications." *Journal of Psychosomatic Research*, 23: 1979, p. 109.

7 Schneider, Mary. "Prenatal stress impact on rhesus monkey learning." University of Wisconsin, 1996.

8 Samuels, Mike and Nancy. *The New Well Pregnancy Book*. Fireside: New York, 1996, p. 149.

9 Ibid., p. 161.

10 Ibid., p. 261.

11 Nuckolls, K., et. al. "Psychosocial assets, life crises and the prognosis of pregnancy." *American Journal of Epidemiology* 95: 1972, p. 431.

12 McCutcheon, Susan. *Revised Edition Natural Childbirth the Bradley Way*. Penguin Group: New York, 1980.

13 Dick-Read, Op. Cit., p. 62-78.

14 Kitzinger, Sheila. *The Complete Book of Pregnancy and Childbirth*. Alfred A. Knopf, Inc.: New York, 1981.

15 Longworth, J.C. "Psychophysical effects of slow stroke back massage in normotensive females." *Adv Nurs Sci* 4: 1982, p. 44-61.

16 Field, T., C. Morrow, C. Valdon, Sl Larson, C. Kuhn, S. Schanberg. "Massage reduces anxiety in child and adolescent psychiatric patients." *Journal of the American Academy of Child and Adolescent Psychiatry*. 31: 1992, p. 125-131.

17 Ironson, G, Field, T, Kumar, A, et al. "Relaxation through massage is associated with decreased distress and increased serotonin levels." Presented at the Academy of Psychosomatic Medicine, 1992.

18 Field, T, Hernandez-Reif, M, Hart, S, et al. University of Miami School of Medicine Touch Research Abstracts, Spring 1997.

19 Juhan, Deane. *Job's Body: A Handbook for Bodywork*. Station Hill Press: New York, 1987, p. 294.

20 Lockhart, Esther. "Massage therapy: mind/body effects on chronic pain patients." Master's Thesis, University of North Texas, Denton, Texas, 1988.

21 Samuels, Op. Cit., p. 160.

22 Arkko, P.J., Pakarinen, A.J., Kari-Koskinen, O. "Effects of whole-body massage on serum protein, electrolyte and hormone concentrations, enzyme activities and hematological parameters." *International Journal of Sports Medicine* 4:1983, p. 265-267.

23 Foldi, M. "Anatomical and physiological basis for physical therapy of lymphedema." *Experientia* 33 (suppl):1978, p. 15-18.

24 Zanolla, R., Monzeglio, C., Balzarini, A., et al. "Evaluation of the results of three different methods of post-mastectomy lymphedema treatment." *J. Surg. Oncol.* 26:1984, p. 210-13.

25 Linde, B. "Dissociation of insulin absorption and blood flow during massage of a subcutaneous injection site." *Diabetes Care* 6:1986, p. 570-574.

26 Fakouri, C., MS, RN and Jones, P., MSN, RN. "Relaxation Rx: slow stroke back rub." *Journal of Gerontological Nursing*, 13(2), February, 1987, p. 32-35.

27 Longworth, Op. Cit, p. 44-61.

28 Juhan, Op. Cit., p. 24.

29 Montagu, Ashley. *Touching: The Human Significance of the Skin*. Harper & Row: New York, 1978, p. 2.

30 Ruegamer, Berstein, Benjamin. "Growth, food, utilization, and thyriod activity in the albino rat as a function of extra handling." *Science*, 120:1954, p. 184-85.

31 Weininger, O., W.J. Mc Clelland, K. Arima. "Gentling and weight gain in the albino rat." *Canadian Journal of Psychology*, 8:1954, p. 147-51.

32 Pauk, J., C. Kuhn, T. Field, S. Schanberg. "The positive effects of tactile versus kinesthetic or vestibular stimulation on neuroendocrine and ODC activity in maternally deprived rat pups." *Life Science*, 39:1986, p. 2081-87.

33 Tapp, J.T., H. Markowitz. "Infant handling: Effects on avoidance learning, brain weight, and cholinesterase activity." *Science*, 140:1963, p. 486-87.

34 Juraska, J.M., W.T. Greenough, C. Elliott, K.J. Mack, R. Berkowitz. "Plasticity in adult rat visual cortex: An examination of several cell populations after differential rearing." *Behavioral and Neural Biology*, 29:1980, p. 157-67.

35 Meaney, M.J., D.H. Aitken, S.R. Bodnoff, L.J. Iny, R.M. Sapolsky. "The effects of postnatal handling on the development of the glucocorticoid receptor systems and stress recovery on the rat." *Progress in Neuropsychopharmacology and Biological Psychiatry*, 7:1985, p. 731-34.

36 Meaney, M.J., D.H. Aitken, S. Sharma, V. Viau, A. Sarrieau. "Neonatal handling alters adrenocortical negative feedback sensitivity and hippocampal type II glucocorticoid receptor binding in the rat." *Neuroendocrinology*, 50:1989, p. 597-604.

37 Denenberg, V.H., GG. Karas. "Interactive effect of age and duration of infantile experience on adult learning." *Psychological Reports*, 7:1960, p. 313-22.

38 Rosen, J. "Dominance behavior as a function of early gentling experience in the albino rats." Master's Thesis, University of Toronto, 1957.

39 Roth, L.L. and Rosenblatt, J.S. "Mammary glands of pregnant rats: development stimulated by licking." *Science*, 264: March, 1996, p. 1403-04.

40 Noble, Elizabeth. *Essential Exercises for The Childbearing Year. Fourth Edition*. New Life Images: Harwich, MA, 1995, p. 147-159.

41 Witt, P.L., MacKinnon, J. "Trager Psychophysical Integration: A method to improve chest mobility of patients with chronic lung disease." *Phys Ther* 66:1986, p. 214-17.

42 Wheeden, A., Scafidi, F., Field, T., et. al. "Massage effects on cocaine-exposed preterm neonates." *J Dev Behav Pediatr* 14:1993, p. 318-22.

43 Flocco, O. "Randomized controlled study of premenstrual symptoms treated with reflexology." *Obstetrics and Gynecology*, 82:1993, p. 906-11.

44 Belluomini, Jenny, Litt, Robin C., Lee, Katheryn, and Katz, Michael. "Acupressure for nausea and vomiting of pregnancy: a randomized, blinded study." *Obstetrics and Gynecology*, 84: 1994, p. 245.

45 Noble, Op Cit., p. 53-80.

46 Unpublished survey of graduates of pregnancy training programs, Somatic Learning Associates, La Jolla, CA, 1994.

47 Ostgaard, H.C., Andersson, G.B.S., et al. "Prevalence of back pain in pregnancy." *Spine*, January 1992, Vol. 17, No. 1, p. 53-55.

48 Artal, R. Friedman, M.J., McNitt-Gray, J.L. "Orthopedic problems in pregnancy." *The Physician and Sportsmedicine*. 18:No. 9, September 1990, p. 93-105.

49 Noble, Op. Cit., p. 54.

50 Artal, Op. Cit., p. 99.

51 Yates, John, PhD. *A Physician's Guide to Therapeutic Massage: Its Physiological Effects and Their Application to Treatment*. Masssage Therapists' Association of British Columbia: Vancouver, BC, Canada, 1990, p. 12.

52 Lockhart, E., Op. Cit.

53 Sunshine, W, Field, T. Quintino, O, et al. "Fibromyalgia benefits from massage therapy and transcutaneous electrical stimulation." *Journal of Clinical Rheumatology*, 2:1996, p. 18-22.

54 Quebec Task Force on Spinal Disorders. "Scientific approach to the assessment and management of activity-related spinal disorders." *Spine*, 12:No. 7, 1987, Supplement 1, p. 524.

55 Yates, Op. Cit., p. 12.

56 Jones, Lawrence H., D.O. *Strain and Counterstrain*. The American Academy of Osteopathy: Newark, OH, 1981.

57 Osborne-Sheets, C. *Deep Tissue Sculpting: A Technical and Artistic Manual for Therapeutic Bodywork Practitioners*. Body Therapy Associates and International Professional School of Bodywork: San Diego, CA, 1990, p. 13-15.

58 Fritz, S. *Fundamentals of Therapeutic Massage*. Mosby/Lifeline: St. Louis, MO, 1995, p. 134-36.

59 Cyriax, J. "Indications for and against deep friction." *Textbook of Orthopaedic Medicine*. Vol. 2 *Treatment by Manipulation, Massage, and Injection. 11th ed.* Bailliere-Tindall: Toronto, Ontario, Canada, 1984.

60 Travell, J.G., M.D., and Simons, D., M.D. *Myofascial Pain and Dysfunction: The Trigger Point Manual, Volume 2*. Williams and Wilkins: Baltimore, 1992, p. 5.

61 Weintraub, M. "Shiatsu, Swedish massage and trigger point suppression in spinal pain syndrome." *American Journal of Pain Management*, 2(2), April 1992, p. 74-78.

62   Noble, Op. Cit., p. 81-146.

63   Simkin, P., P.T. "Reducing pain and enhancing progress in labor: a guide to nonpharmacologic methods for maternity caregivers." *Birth* 22:3, September 1995, p. 162.

64   Jordan, Sandra. *Yoga for Pregnancy: Safe and Gentle Stretches*. St. Martin's Press: New York, 1988.

65   Dancing Through Pregnancy, Inc., Pre/postnatal health and fitness programs, (800) 442-9034.

66   Noble, Op. Cit., p. 19-52.

67   "Marie Osmond's Exercises for Mothers-to-Be" (video), Elizabeth Noble, P.T. New Life Images, Harwich, MA (508) 432-8040.

68   Samuels, Op. Cit., p. 103.

69   Hanna, Thomas. *Somatics: Reawakening the Mind's Control of Movement, Flexibility, and Health*. Addison-Wesley: Menlo Park, CA, 1988, p. 27

70   Noble, Op. Cit., p. 65-68, 83-88, 151-159.

71   Samuels, Op. Cit, p. 19.

72   Birch, E., "The experience of touch received during labor." *Journal of Nurse-Midwifery*, 31, p. 270-75.

73   Milner, I., "Water baths for pain relief in labor." *Nursing Times*, January 6, 1988, p. 38-40.

74   Lesser, M., and Keane, V. *Nurse-Patient Relationships in a Hospital Maternity Setting*. Mosby: St. Louis, MO, 1956.

75   Field, T., Hernandez-Reif, M., Taylor, S., Quintino, O. Touch Research Institute, University of Miami School of Medicine and Iris Burman, Educating hands School of Massage Therapy. *Journal of Psychosomatic Obstetrics and Gynecology*, (in press, 1998).

76   Saltenis, I. "Physical touch and nursing support in labor." Unpublished Master's Thesis, Yale University, New Haven, CT, 1962.

77   Klaus, M., et.al. "Effects of social support during parturition on maternal-infant morbidity." *British Medical Journal* 293:1986, p. 585-87.

78   Kennell,J., et al. "Medical intervention: the effect of social support during labor." *Pediatric Research* 23:1988, p. 211.

79   Hodnett, E. and Osborn, R. "A randomized trial of the effects of monitrice support during labor: mothers' views two to four weeks postpartum." *Birth* 16(4):1989, p. 177-84.

80   Klaus, M.H., M.D., Kennell, J.H., M.D., and Klaus, P.H., M.Ed., C.S.W. *Mothering the Mother: How a Doula Can Help You Have a Shorter, Easier, and Healthier Birth*. Addison-Wesley: Reading, MA, 1993, p. 51.

81   Green, J.M., Coupland, V.A., and Kitzinger, J.V. "Expectations, experiences and psychological outcomes of childbirth." *Birth*: 17:1990, p. 15-24.

82   Simkin, P. "Just another day in a woman's life? Part 1. Women's long-term perceptions of their first birth experience." *Birth*: 18:1991, p. 203-210.

83   Harlow, H.F., M.K. Harlow, E.W. Hansen. "The maternal affectional system of rhesus monkeys." In: Reingold (ed), *Maternal Behavior in Mammals*, Wiley: New York, 1963.

84   Settle, Faustine. "Muzica, Da? My Experience in a Romanian Orphanage." *Massage Therapy Journal*, Fall, 1991, p. 64-72.

85 Denenberg, V.H., E.E. Whimbey. "Behavior of adult rats is modified by the experiences their mothers had as infants." *Science*, 142:1963, p. 1192-93.

86 Montague, Op. Cit., p. 77-78

87 Goldsmith, E.I. and Moor-Janowski, J. (eds.), "Early somatosensory deprivation as an ontogenetic process in the abnormal development of the brain and behavior." In: *Medical Primatology*, S. Karger: New York, 1971, p. 1-20.

88 Prescott, J.II. "Body pleasure and the origins of violence." *The Futurist*, April 1975, p. 64-65.

89 Rubin, R. *Maternal Identity and the Maternal Experience*. Springer Publishing: New York, 1984.

90 Rubin, R. "Maternal tasks in pregnancy." *Maternity Child Nursing Journal*, 4:1975, p. 143-53.

91 Rubin, R. "Maternal touch." *Nursing Outlook*, Vol. 11, 1963, p. 828-31.

92 Field, T., S. Schanberg et al. "Tactile/kinesthetic stimulation effects on preterm neonates." *Pediatr* 77/5:1986, p. 654-58

93 Pediatric Roundtable #10, "The many facets of touch. The foundation of experience: Its importance through life, with initial emphasis for infants and young children. " Ed: C. Caldwell Brown, Johnson and Johnson: Skillman, New Jersey, 1984.

94 Pediatric Roundtable #14, "Advances in touch: New implications in human development." Ed: N. Gunzenhauser, Johnson and Johnson: Skillman, New Jersey, 1990.

95 Rausch, P.B. "Effects of tactile and kinesthetic stimulation on premature infants." *J Obstet Gynecol Neonatal Nurs*, 10:1981, p. 34-37.

96 Rice, R. "The effects of the Rice sensorimotor stimulation treatment on the development of high risk infants." Birth Defects Original Article Series, 15:1979, A.R. Liss: New York, p. 7-26.

97 Scafidi, F.A., T.M. Field, S.M. Schanberg, S.R. Bauer, K. Tucci, J. Roberts, C. Morrow and C.M. Kuhn. "Massage stimulates growth in preterm infants: A replication." *Infant Behavior and Develop*, 13:1990, p. 167-88.

98 Scafidi, F.A., T.M Field, S.M. Schanberg, S.R. Bauer, N. Vega-Lahr, R. Garcia, J. Poirier, G. Nystrom, C.M. Kuhn. "Effects of tactile/kinesthetic stimulation on the clinical course and sleep/wake behavior of preterm neonates." *Infant Behavior and Develop*, 9:1986, p. 91-105.

99 Solkoff, N., S. Yaffe, D. Weintraub, B. Blase. "Effects of handling on the subsequent development of premature infants." *Develop Psychology*, 1:1969, p. 765-68.

100 White, J.L., R.C. Labarba. " The effects of tactile and kinesthetic stimulation on neonatal development in the premature infant." *Develop Psychobiology*, 6:1976, p. 569-77.

101 Field, T., Gruzzle, N., Scafidi, F., et al. "Massage therapy for infants of depressed mothers." *Infant Behavior and Development*, 1995.

102 Anderson, G., Marks, E., and Wahlberg, V. "Kangaroo care for premature infants." *American Journal of Nursing* 7, July, p. 806-07.

103 Certification in infant massage instruction is offered by:
International Association of Infant Massage, see Resources appendix.
Rice Infant Sensorimotor Stimulation, see Resources appendix

104 Simkin, P. "The experience of maternity in a woman's life." *Journal of Obstetrical and gynocological Nursing*, March/April, 1996, p. 247-252.

105 Hufnagel, V., M.D. "Medical basis for using massage after surgery." *Massage Magazine* #17, Dec-Jan/1988-89, p. 21.

106 Fritz, Op. Cit., p. 87-88.

107 Oleson, T, Flocco, W. "Randomized controlled study of premenstrual symptoms treated with ear, hand, and foot reflexology." *Obstetrics and Gynecology*, 82 (6), December 1993, p. 906-1110.

108 Noble, Op. Cit., p. 88-106.

Chapter 2, Guidelines and Precautions for Pre- and Perinatal Massage Therapy

1 Gilbert, Elizabeth Stepp and Harmon, Judith Smith. *Manual of High Risk Pregnancy and Delivery*. St. Louis, MO: Mosby-Year Book, Inc., 1993, p. 40.

2 Noble, Elizabeth. *Essential Exercises for The Childbearing Year. Fourth Edition*. New Life Images: Harwich, MA, 1995, p. 44.

3 Ibid., p. 44.

4 Ibid., p. 128.

5 Samuels, Mike and Nancy. *The New Well Pregnancy Book*. Fireside: New York, 1996, p. 145.

6 Juhan, Deane. *Job's Body: A Handbook for Bodywork*. Station Hill Press: New York, 1987, p. 208-209.

7 Osborne-Sheets, Carole. "Pre- and Perinatal Massage Therapy," see Resources appendix.

8 Knott, M. and Voss, D. *Proprioceptive Neuromuscular Facilitation*. Harper & Row: New York, 1956.

9 Upledger, John E., D.O. and Vredervogd, D., M.F.A. *Craniosacral Therapy*. Eastland Press: Seattle, WA, 1983.

10 Cyriax, J. and Coldham, M. *The Textbook of Orthopaedic Medicine Treatment by Manipulation, Massage, and Injection*, Vol. 2, Ed. 11, Bailliere, Tindall: East Sussex, England, 1984.

11 Osborne-Sheets, C. *Deep Tissue Sculpting: A Technical and Artistic Manual for Therapeutic Bodywork Practitioners*. Body Therapy Associates and International Professional School of Bodywork: San Diego, CA, 1990.

12 Maupin, Edward W., Ph.D. *The Structural Metaphor*. International Professional School of Bodywork, San Diego, CA, 1993.

13 Rolf, Ida P., Ph.D. *Rolfing, The Integration of Human Structures*. Harper & Row: New York, 1977.

14 Maupin, Edward, Ph.D. *The Genie in the Bottle: Psychology for Bodyworkers*. International Professional School of Bodywork, San Diego, CA 1992.

15 Bogardus, Stephen. "Aunty Margaret Revisited: Lomilomi Massage and Hawaiian Healing Arts Master." *Massage Magazine*, Vol. 1, #6, 1986.

16 Tappan, Francis M., Ed.D. *Healing Massage Techniques: Holistic, Classic, and Emerging Methods*. Appleton & Lange: East Norwalk, CT, 1988.

17 Fritz, S. *Fundamentals of Therapeutic Massage*. Mosby/Lifeline: St. Louis, MO, 1995.

18 "Dr. Milton Trager, An Exclusive Interview." *Massage Magazine*, #15, Aug/Sept, 1988.

19 Osborne-Sheets, Carole. "Deep Tissue/Passive Movement Blends," see Resources appendix.

20 Mower, Melissa. "Exclusive Interview, Carole Osborne-Sheets, Teacher, Bodyworker, Author." *Massage Magazine #46*, Nov/Dec, 1993, p. 44-52.

21 Osborne-Sheets, Carole. "Deep Tissue/Passive Movement Blends," see Resources appendix.

22 Jones, Lawrence H., D.O. *Strain and Counterstrain*. American Academy of Osteopathy: Newark, OH, 1981.

23 Anderson, Dale L., M.D. *Muscle Pain Relief in 90 Seconds: The Fold and Hold Method*. Chronimed Publishing: Minneapolis, MN, 1995.

24 Anderson, Bob. *Stretching*. Shelter Publications: Bolinas, CA, 1980.

25 Kaptchuck, Ted. *The Web that Has No Weaver*. Congdon & Weed: Chicago, IL, 1983.

26 Ebner, Maria. *Connective Tissue Manipulations: Theory and Therapeutic Application*. Krieger Publishing: Malabar, FL, 1985.

27 Marquardt, Hanne. *Reflex Zone Therapy of the Feet: Textbook for Therapists*. Healing Arts Press: Rochester, VT, 1984.

28 Travell, J.G., M.D. and Simons, D.G., M.D. *Myofascial Pain and Dysfunction: The Trigger Point Manual*. Vol. 1 & 2, Williams & Wilkins: Baltimore, MD, 1983.

29 Courses offered at International Professional School of Bodywork, see Resources appendix.

30 Fritz, Op. Cit.

31 Tappan, Op. Cit.

32 Gilbert, Op. Cit., p. 264.

33 Ibid., p. 415-416.

34 Ibid., p. 416.

35 Jefferies, Walltam S., and Felix Bochner. "Thromboembolism and its management in pregnancy." *Med J Australia*, Vol.155, August, 1991, p. 253.

36 Alexander, Doug. "Deep vein thrombisis and massage therapy." *Massage Therapy Journal 32:2*, Spring 1993, p. 58.

37 Jefferies, Op. Cit., p. 253.

38 Gibbs, N.M. "Venous thrombosis of the lower limbs with particular reference to bed-rest." *Br J Surg* 1957: 45, p. 209-36.

39 Jefferies, Op. Cit., p. 253.

40 Gilbert, Op. Cit., p. 352.

41 Alexander, Op. Cit., p. 58.

42 Ohaski, Wataru and Hoover, Mary. *Natural Childbirth the Eastern Way*. Ballantine Books: New York, p. 10.

43 Simkin, P., Whalley, J., and Keppler, A. *Pregnancy, Childbirth, and the Newborn*. Meadowbrook Press: New York, 1991, p. 87.

44 Rich, Laurie, A. *When Pregnancy Isn't Perfect*. Dutton: New York, 1991, p. 5.

45   Gilbert, Op. Cit., p. 266.

46   Ibid., p. 465.

47   Rothman, Barbara Katz. *Encyclopedia of Childbearing*. Oryx Press: Phoenix, AZ, 1993, p. 111.

48   Ibid., p. 384.

49   Gilbert, Op. Cit., p. 323.

50   Ibid., p. 330.

51   Samuels, Op Cit., p. 290.

52   Rich, Op. Cit., p. 47-48.

53   Samuels, Op. Cit., p. 233.

54   Ibid., p. 251-252.

55   Rich, Op. Cit., p. 75-76.

56   Gilbert, Op. Cit., p. 180.

57   Rich, Op. Cit., p. 62.

58   Samuels, Op. Cit., p. 240.

59   Gilbert, Op. Cit., p. 25-37.

60   Samuels, Op. Cit., p. 240.

61   Rothman, Op. Cit., p. 395-399.

62   Boyer, D. and Fine, D. "Sexual abuse as a factor in adolescent pregnancy and child maltreatment." *Family Planning Perspectives*, 24:1992, p. 4-19.

63   Simkin, Penny, Whalley, Janet, and Keppler, Ann. *Pregnancy, Childbirth, and the Newborn*. Meadowbrook Press: New York, 1991, p. 35.

64   Gilbert, Op. Cit., p. 266.

65   Samuels, Op. Cit., p. 240.

66   Rich, Op. Cit., p. 214-217.

67   Gilbert, Op. Cit., p. 180.

68   Ibid., p. 185-186.

69   Ibid., p. 188-189.

70   Ibid., p. 219.

71   Ibid., p. 220.

72   Ibid., p. 237-238.

73   Ibid., p. 238.

74   Ibid., p. 252.

75   Ibid., p. 250.

76 Rich, Op. Cit., p. 191.

77 Gilbert, Op. Cit., p. 269.

78 Ibid., p. 277.

79 Ibid., p. 34.

80 Simkin, Penny, P.T. "Overcoming the Legacy of Childhood Sexual Abuse: The Role of Caregivers and Childbirth Educators." *Birth*, 19.4, Dec., 1992, p. 224-225.

81 Evans, A. "Childhood sexual abuse, prematurity, and neonatal medical problems," presented at the Pre- and Perinatal Psychology Association of North America Congress in Amherst, MA, 1989.

82 Gilbert, Op. Cit., p. 160.

Chapter 3, Trimester Recommendations

1 Verralls, Sylvia. *Anatomy & Physiology Applied to Obstetrics. Third Edition*. Churchill Livingstone: New York, 1993, p. 181.

2 Simkin, P., Whalley, J., Keppler, A. *Pregnancy Childbirth and the Newborn: The Complete Guide*. Meadowbrook Press: New York, 1991, p. 26.

3 Samuels, Mike and Nancy. *The New Well Pregnancy Book*. Fireside: New York, 1996, p. 46-56.

4 Jimenez, Sherry. *The Pregnant Woman's Comfort Guide*. Avery Publishing Group, Inc.: Garden City Park, New York, 1992, p. 91-92.

5 Profet, Margie. *Protecting Your Baby-to-Be*. Addison-Wesley: New York, 1995.

6 Baldwin, Rahima and Palmarini Richardson, Terra. *Pregnant Feelings: Developing Trust in Birth*. Celestial Arts: Berkeley, CA, 1986.

7 Noble, Elizabeth. *Essential Exercises for The Childbearing Year. Fourth Edition*. New Life Images: Harwich, MA, 1995.

8 Bing, Elizabeth. *Elizabeth Bing's Guide to Moving Through Pregnancy*. Noonday Press: New York, 1991.

9 Klein Olkin, Sylvia. *Positive Pregnancy Fitness*. Avery Publishing Group: New York, 1987.

10 Tisserand, Maggie. *Aromatherapy for Women*. Thorson's Publishers, Inc.: New York, 1985.

11 Belluomini, Jenny, MSN, Litt, Robin C., MSN, Lee, Kathryn A., RN, PhD, and Katz, Michael, MD. "Acupressure for nausea and vomiting of pregnancy: a randomized, blinded study." *Obstetrics & Gynecology*. 84:1994, p. 245.

12 Myers, Thomas W. "The 'anatomy trains." *Journal of Bodywork and Movement Therapies*. Vol 1 & 2, Jan. 1997, p. 91-101.

13 Gilbert, Elizabeth Stepp and Harmon, Judith Smith. *Manual of High Risk Pregnancy and Delivery*. Mosby-Year Book, Inc.: St. Louis, MO, 1993, p. 16.

14 Noble, Op. Cit., p. 107-117.

15 Osborne-Sheets, Carole. *Deep Tissue Sculpting: A Technical and Artistic Manual for Therapeutic Bodywork Practitioners*. Body Therapy Associates and International Professional School of Bodywork: San Diego, CA, 1990.

16 Leduc, Marie, R.N. "Stretch marks: striae gravidarum." In: *Encyclopedia of Childbearing: Critical Perspectives*. The Oryx Press: Phoenix, Arizona, 1993, p 385.

17 Lesko, Wendy & Matthew. *The Maternity Sourcebook*. Warner Books: New York, 1984, p. 164.

18 *Planning for Pregnancy, Birth, and Beyond*. American College of Obstetrics and Gynecology, 1990, p. 130.

19 Rich, Laurie A. *When Pregnancy Isn't Perfect*. Dutton: New York, 1991, p. 76.

20 Ibid., p. 283-310.

21 Noble, Op. Cit., p. 147-151.

22 Gilbert, Op. Cit., p. 17-18.

23 Noble, Op. Cit., p. 210-213.

24 Campbell, Leslie Kirk. *Journey Into Motherhood*. Riverhead Books: New York, 1996.

25 Medcom Video. "Massage for pregnancy and labor," see Resources appendix.

26 Chester, Laura. *Cradle and All: Women Writers on Pregnancy and Birth*. Faber and Faber: Boston, MA, 1989.

27 Otten, Charlotte, Editor. *The Book of Birth Poetry*. Bantam Books: New York, 1995.

28 Simkin, *Pregnancy, Childbirth, and the Newborn*, Op. Cit., p. 91.

29 Varassi, H., et. al. "Effects of physical activity on maternal plasma beta-endorphin levels and perception of labor pain. *Am. J. of Ob/Gyn.* #160 (March, 1989), p. 707.

30 Medvin, Jeannine O'Brien. *Prenatal Yoga and Natural Birth*. Freestone Publishing Co.: Albion, CA, 1978.

31 Markowitz, E. & Brainen, H. *Baby Dance: A Comprehensive Guide to Prenatal and Postpartum Exercise*. Prentice Hall, Inc.: Englewood Cliffs, NJ, 1980.

32 Olkin, Sylvia Klein, Op. Cit.

33 Holstein, Barbara B. *Shaping Up For a Healthy Pregnancy*. Life Enhancement Publications: Champaign, IL, 1988.

34 "Everymom's Prenatal Exercise and Relaxation Video." Quantum Video (805) 962-0871.

35 Gilbert, Op. Cit., p. 16.

36 Noble, Op. Cit., p. 48-50.

37 Ibid, p. 39-48.

38 Rolf, Ida, Ph.D. *Rolfing: The Integration of Human Structures*. Harper & Row: New York, 1977, p. 101-121.

39 Samuels, Op. Cit., p. 248-250.

40 Kitzinger, Sheila. *Celebration of Birth*. ICEA/Pennypress: Minneapolis, MN, 1986, p. 8.

41 Maybruck, P. *Pregnancy and Dreams*. Jeremy P. Tarcher, Inc.: Los Angeles, CA, 1989.

42 Gaskin, Ina May. *Spiritual Midwifery*. The Book Publishing Company: Summertown, TN, 1977.

43 Simkin, Penny. "Overcoming the legacy of childhood sexual abuse." Midwifery Today Conference workshop presentation materials, March, 1997.

44 Sutton, Jean and Scott, Pauline. *Understanding and Teaching Optimal Foetal Positioning*. Birth Concepts. New Zealand, 1996, p. 18 and 29.

45 Wine, Zhenya A. "Massage for varicose veins." *Massage Magazine*, #66, March/April, 97, p. 133-135.

46 Stephens, Suzanne. "Body work and childbirth, proven wonders." *International Journal of Childbirth Education*, Vol. 12, No. 4, December 1997, p. 20-21.

47 Novak, Janice. *Enhancing Lamaze Techniques: Exercise Book for Pregnancy, Birth, and Recovery*, Body Press (Price, Stern, Sloan), 1988.

48 Avery , M.D. and Burket, B.A. "Effect of perineal massage on incidence of episiotomy and perineal laceration in a nurse-midwifery service." *Journal of Nurse-Midwifery*. 31(3), May-June, 1986, p. 128-34.

49 Noble, Op. Cit., p. 58.

50 Simkin, Penny. *The Birth Partner*. Harvard Common Press: Boston, MA, 1989, p. 15.

51 Mynaugh, Patricia A. "The effectiveness of prenatal health practices and two instructional educational methods on labor and delivery: a case study of perineal massage." *Dissertation Abstracts International*, #8902979. University Microfilms, Inc.: Ann Arbor, MI, 1988.

52 Simkin. *The Birth Partner*, Op Cit., p. 16-17.

53 Lieberman, Adrienne B. *Easing Labor Pain*. Doubleday & Company: New York, 1987, p. 57-70.

54 Simkin, *Pregnancy, Childbirth, and the Newborn*, Op. Cit., p 105-112.

55 Kitzinger, Sheila. *The Complete Book of Pregnancy and Childbirth*. Alfred A. Knopf, Inc.: New York, 1981, p. 165-172.

56 McCafferty, Tracy Games. "Labor of love." *Yoga Journal*, Jan/Feb, 1997, p. 85-92.

57 Medcom Video. "Massage for Pregnancy and Labor," see Resources appendix.

58 View Video. "Infant Massage: The Power of Touch," see Resources appendix.

59 Schneider McClure, Vimala. *Infant Massage: A Handbook for Loving Parents*. Bantam Books: New York, 1989.

60 International Association of Infant Massage Instructors, see Resources appendix.

61 Gilbert, Op. Cit., p. 601-606.

62 Simkin, *Pregnancy, Childbirth and the Newborn*, Op Cit., p. 167-169.

Chapter 4, Labor and Birth Facilitation

1 Samuels, Mike and Nancy. *The New Well Pregnancy Book*. Fireside: New York, 1996, p. 260.

2 Pajntar, M. "Psychosomatic disturbances in the course of labor." In: Prill, H., *Advances in Psychosomatic Obstetrics and Gynecology*. Springer-Verlag, 1982.

3 Dick-Read, Grantly, M.D. *Childbirth Without Fear*, Fifth Edition. Harper & Row: NY, 1984, p. 67.

4 Harper, Barbara, R.N. *Gentle Birth Choices*. Healing Arts Press: Rochester, VT, 1994, p. 51-59.

5   Goer, Henci. *Obstetrical Myths Versus Research Realities: A Guide to the Medical Literature.* Bergin & Garvey: Westport, CT, 1995, p. 331-347.

6   Granden, A., "Maternal anxiety and obstetric complications." *Journal of Psychosomatic Research,* 23: 1979, p. 109.

7   Kitzinger, Sheila. *The Complete Book of Pregnancy and Childbirth.* Alfred A. Knopf: New York, 1981, p. 236-240.

8   Simkin, Penny. "Non-pharmacological methods of pain relief for labor." Midwifery Today Conference workshop presentation, March, 1997.

9   Ibid.

10 Craig, J. "Emotional aspects of pain." In: P. Wall & R. Melzack (Eds.), *Textbook of Pain.* Churchill Livingstone: New York, 1989, p. 220-230.

11 Simkin, Penny. "Overcoming the legacy of childhood sexual abuse: the role of caregivers and childbirth educators." *Birth* 19:4 Dec. 1992, p. 224-225.

12 Dick-Read, Op. Cit., p. 196-203.

13 McCutcheon, Susan. *Revised Edition Natural Childbirth the Bradley Way.* Penguin Group, 1986.

14 American Society for Psycho-Prophylaxis in Obstetrics, Inc. (ASPO). 1200 19th St., NW #300, Washington, D.C. 20036-2422. (800) 368-4404. (Lamaze Method.)

15 Kitzinger, Op. Cit. p. 162.

16 Bonica, J. "The nature of the pain of parturition." In: Bonica, JJ, MacDonald, JS, (Eds.) *Principles and Practice of Obstetric Analgesia and Anesthesia.* 2nd ed. Williams & Wilkins: Baltimore, MD, 1995, p. 243-273.

17 Lieberman, Adrienne B., *Easing Labor Pain: The Complete Guide to Achieving a More Comfortable and Rewarding Birth,* Doubleday & Company, Inc: Garden City, NY, 1987, p. 92-103 & 133-156.

18 Thorp, JA, Hu DH, Albin RM, et al. "Effect of intrpartum epidural analgesia on nulliparous labor; a randomized prospective trial." *Am J Obstet Gynecol* 1993; 169, p. 851.

19 Avard, D.M. and Nimrod C.M. "Risks and benefits of obstetric epidural analgesia; a review." *Birth* 12(4):1985, p. 215-225.

20 Thorp, James A, MD. "Weighing the benefits of epidural analgesia during labor." *Contemporary Ob/Gyn,* April 1997, p. 95-106.

21 Dickersin, K. "Pharmacologic control of pain during labour." In: Chalmers, I., Enkin, M. and Kiere, M. (Eds.) *Effective Care in Pregnancy and Childbirth.* Oxford University Press, 1995, p. 913.

22 Simkin, Penny. "Stress, pain and catecholamines in labor. Part 1. A review of the literature." *Birth* 13:1986, p. 227-233.

23 Sepkoske CM, Lester BM, Ostheimer GW, and Brazelton TB. "The effects of maternal epidural anesthesia on neonatal behavior during the first month." *Dev Med Child Neurol* 1992; 34, p. 1072-1080.

24 Dickersin, Op. Cit., p. 115.

25 Simkin, Penny, P.T. "Reducing pain and enhancing progress in labor: a guide to nonpharmacologic methods for maternity caregivers." *Birth* 22:3, September, 1995, p. 161.

26 Simkin, Penny. "Non-pharmacological methods of pain relief during labor." In: Chalmers, Enkin, and Kerise (Eds.). *Effective Care in Pregnancy and Birth, Vol II*. Oxford University Press, 1989.

27 Melzack, R.D. *The Puzzle of Pain*. Basic Books: New York, 1973.

28 Harper, Op. Cit., p. 14.

29 Jones, C. *Mind Over Labor*. Penquin Books: New York, 1987, p. 21-23.

30 Hale, Marie Fellenstein and Chalmers, Liz. *The Childbirth Kit: Ideas and Images to Help You Through Labor*. Swanstone Press, 1994.

31 Harper, Op. Cit., p. 169-186.

32 Green, J.M., Coupland, V.A. and Kitzinger, J.V. "Expectations, experiences, and psychological outcomes of childbirth." *Birth*: 17:1990, p. 15-24.

33 Caldeyro-Barcia, R. "The effect of position changes on the intensity and frequency of uterine contractions during labor." *American Journal of Obstetrics and Gynecology* 80:1960, p. 284.

34 Simkin, Op. Cit., *Birth* 22:3, p. 162-167.

35 Cammu H, Clasen K, Van Wettern L. "Is having a warm bath during labour useful?" *Acta Obstet Gynecol Scand* 1994: 73; p. 468-472.

36 Harper, Op. Cit., p. 134-135.

37 Khomis, Y., Shaala, S., Damarawy, H., Romia, A., and Toppozada, M. "Effect of heat on uterine contractions during normal labor." *Int. J gynaecol Obstetric* 21:1983, p. 491-493.

38 McNiven, P., Hodnett, E., O'Brien-Pallas, L. "Supporting women in labor: a work sampling study of the activities of labor and delivery nurses." *Birth* 19:1992, p. 3-8.

39 Harper, Op. Cit., p. 190-192.

40 Jones, Op. Cit., p. 142-143.

41 Cogan, R. "Backache in prepared childbirth." *Birth and the Family Journal* 3:2:1976, p. 75.

42 El Halta, Valerie. "Posterior labor: A pain in the back! Its prevention and cure." *Midwifery Today*.

43 Simkin, *The Birth Partner*, Op. Cit., p. 111.

44 Simkin, Op Cit. *Birth* 22:3, p. 162.

45 Jones, Op. Cit., p. 60-62.

46 Golay, Jan, Vedam, Saraswathi, and Sorger, Leo. "The squatting position of the second stage of Labor: effects on labor and on maternal and fetal well-being." *Birth* 20:2 June 1993, p. 73-78.

47 "News." *Birth* 24:3 September, 1997, p. 199.

48 Griffin, Nancy. "Avoiding an episiotomy." *Mothering*, #75, Summer 1995, p. 57.

61 "News." *Birth* 24:3 September, 1997, p. 199.

Chapter 5, Postpartum Bodywork

1 Lim, Robin. "Postpartum Practices throughout the world." *Mothering*, Spring 1993, p. 86-87.

2   Kitzinger, Sheila. *Ourselves as Mothers: the Universal Experience of Motherhood.* Addison-Wesley Publishing Company: New York, p. 176-186.

3   Kitzinger, Sheila. *The Year After Childbirth.* Charles Schribner's Sons: New York, 1994, p. 30-31.

4   MacArthur, C., Lesi M., Knox EG, and Crawford JS. "Epidural anaesthesia and long-term bachache after childbirth." *British Medical Journal*, 301:1990, p. 9-12.

5   Lieberman, Adrienne. *Easing Labor Pain: The Complete Guide to Achieving a More Comfortable and Rewarding Birth.* Doubleday and Company: New York, 1987, p. 129-130.

6   ASPO/Lamaze. *Special Report on Breastfeeding.* Vol 1, #1, October, 1997.

7   ASPO/Lamaze. *Special Report on Breastfeeding.* Vol 2, April, 1998.

8   Righard, M.D., Lennart and Margaret Alade, R.N., BSC, MS. "Delivery self-attachment," *Lancet*, 1990, 336d, p. 105-107.

9   Sims, C.I. "Kangaroo Care." *Mothering* Fall, 1988.

10 "Epidurals: root cause of serious problems." *Midwifery Today*, Autumn, 1997, p. 64.

11 Lieberman, Op. Cit., p. 238.

12 Samuels, Mike and Nancy. *The New Well Pregnancy Book.* Fireside: New York, 1996, p. 346.

13 Kitzinger, *The Year After Childbirth*, Op. Cit., p. 33.

14 Kehoe, C. *The Cesarean Experience.* Appleton-Century-Crofts: New York, 1981, p. 196.

15 Samuels, Op. Cit., p. 370.

16 "Psychiatric issues of the postpartum period." *Currents in Affective Illness: Literature Review and Commentary*, Oct, 1992, p. 5.

17 Kirschenbaum, S. "More than Blue." *Mothering*, Spring, 1995, p. 79.

18 "Psychiatric issues of the postpartum period," Op. Cit., p. 7.

19 Field T., Sandberg D., Garcia R., Vega-Lahr N., Goldstein S., Guy L. "Pregnancy problems, postprartum depression, and early mother-infant interactions." *Dev Psychol* 1985:21, p. 1152-1156.

20 Samuels, Op. Cit., p. 406-408.

21 Harrison, Helen. *The Premature Baby Book.* St. Martin's Press: New York, 1983, p. 9.

22 Kitzinger, *The Year After Childbirth*, Op. Cit., p. 146.

23 Blake Gleeson, P., and Pauls, J. "Carpal tunnel syndrome: during pregnancy and lactation." *PT Magazine*, September, 1993, p. 52-54.

24 Jeffries, J. & Bochner, F. "Thromboembolism and its management in pregnancy." *The Medical Journal of Australia*, Vol. 155, August 19, 1991, p. 253-258.

25 Ibid.

26 Kirschenbaum, Op. Cit., p. 79.

27 Gonzalez, Dona Hermila and Naoli Vinaver. "Massage Techniques from Mexico." Workshop presentation at Midwifery Today conference, March, 1997.

28 Kitzinger, *The Year After Childbirth*, Op. Cit., p. 123-128.

29 Lesko, Wendy & Matthew. *The Maternity Sourcebook*. Warner Books: New York, 1984, p. 163.

30 Lieberman, Op. Cit., p. 231-232.

31 Fitch, Pamela. "The case for breast massage." *Massage Therapy Journal*, Winter 1998, Vol. 36, No. 4, p. 64-78.

32 Polseno Crawford, Dianne. "Why don't we do breast massage?" *Massage Therapy Journal*, Winter 1998, Vol. 36, No. 4, p. 95-106.

33 DeMarco, Carolyn. "How to handle the not-so-joyful parts of pregnancy." *Today's Health*, April/May, 1990. p. 15-18.

34 Noble, Elizabeth. *Essential Exercises for The Childbearing Year*. Fourth Edition. New Life Images: Harwich, MA, 1995, p. 88-105.

35 Myers, Thomas. "Poise: Psoas-Piriformis Balance." *Massage Magazine*, #72, March/April 98, p. 72-83.

36 Chikly, Bruno, MD and Chikly, Alaya, CMT. "Applications of pre-and post-surgical lymphatic drainage therapy." *Massage and Bodywork*, Summer/Fall, 1997, p. 64-67.

37 Javril, Marci and Hufnagel, Vicki, M.D. "Post-surgical massage for female disorders." *Massage Magazine*, Issue 17, Dec/Jan, 1988 89, p. 215.

38 Noble, Op. Cit., p. 203.

39 Chickly, Op. Cit., p. 65.

40 Hufnagel, V., M.D. "Medical basis for using massage after surgery." *Massage Magazine*, Issue 17, Dec/Jan, 1988-89, p. 21.

41 "Facts about sudden infant death syndrome and reducing the risks for SIDS." The Sudden Infant Death Syndrome Alliance, 1994.

42 Rosenberg, Jennifer. "Slings: Rediscovering mother's mobility." *Midwifery Today*, Number 44, Winter 1997, p. 21.

43 Rosenberg, Jennifer. "Slings: Rediscovering mother's mobility, Part 2." *Midwifery Today*. Number 45, Spring, 1998, p. 27-68.

Resources Appendix:

Products:

Baby Bundler. 17310 SW Bryant, Lake Oswego, OR 97035. (800) 253-3502.

Baby Wrap. P.O. Box 100584, Dept. M, Denver, CO 80250-0584.

Contoured bodyCushion®. Available through Body Therapy Associates, (858) 748 8827, (800) 586 8322, or Body Support Systems, Inc., P.O. Box 337, Ashland, OR 97520, (541) 488-1172.

"Massage for Pregnancy & Labor." Instructional video for partners with primary technical consultation provided to producer Med-Com, Inc. by Carole Osborne-Sheets. Available through Body Therapy Associates, (858) 748-8827, (800) 586-8322.

Maya Wrap. 1541 S. 109th St., Omaha, NE 68144. (888) Maya Wrap (628 2872), (www.top.net/mayawrap).

NoJo Sling. 22942 Arroyo Vista Rancho, Santa Margarita, CA 92688. (800) 440-NoJo; Fax: (714) 858-9686; (info@nojo.com) (http://www.nojo.com/).

Over the Shoulder Baby Holder. C.D.M., P.O. Box 635, San Clemente, CA 92674-0635. (800) 637-9426. http://www.babyholder.com/.

Pain Medications Preference Scale, developed by Penny Simkin. Available from Childbirth Graphics, Product #JH 52553. P.O. Box 21207, Waco, TX 76702-1207. (800) 299-3366.

Prenatal support belt, REENIE Maternity Belt. Leading Lady, Inc. 24050 Commerce Park, Beachwood, OH 44122. (216) 464-5490, for stores in your area.

Small prenatal support pillows for the abdomen and for shifting the uterus off the vena cava. Available through Body Therapy Associates, (858) 748-8827, (800) 586 8322 or Spinal Care Systems, (800) 877-6953.

Tilt top massage table models:
Golden Ratio Woodworks, P.O. Box 297, Emigrant Montana 59027, (800) 345-1129.
Living Earth Crafts, 600 East Todd Rd., Santa Rosa, CA 95407 (800) 358-8292.

Wedges for semireclining foundation: 16" wide, #1613; 20" wide, #2013, Orthopedic Physical Therapy Products, (800) 367-7393.

Education:

Aston Patterning®. Bodywork, movement coaching, ergonomics, and fitness trainings. The Aston Training Center, P.O. Box 3568, Incline Village, NV 89450. (702) 831-8228. AstonPat@aol.com.

Association of Labor Assistants and Childbirth Educators (ALACE). P.O. Box 382724, Cambridge, MA 02238, 617-441-2500. World Wide Web: http://www.alace.org.

Carole Osborne Sheets: Body Therapy Associates, 11650 Iberia Place, #137, San Diego, CA, CA (858) 748-8827, (800) 586-8322, www.bodytherapyassociates.com, cos9@aol.com
> *Pre- and Perinatal Massage Therapy*: 32-hour certification in advanced techniques (deep tissue, passive movement, neuromuscular, reflexive, and other soft tissue methods) for pregnant, laboring, and postpartum women; workshops throughout North America.
> *Deep Tissue Passive Movement Blends Introduction*: two days basic instruction in non-intrusive soft tissue work simultaneously performing deep myofascial techniques with rhythmic mobilizations; intensive body mechanics guidance; workshops throughout North America.
> *Introduction to Somatoemotional Integration*: two-day introduction to working with the feeling body to create more balance between the physical, emotional, and intellectual body centers.

Somatoemotional Integration: 60-hour certificate program at International Professional School of Bodywork (IPSB), San Diego, CA. (Prerequisites.)

Doulas of North America (DONA). 1100 23rd Ave. E., Seattle, WA 98112. (206) 324-5440.

International Association of Infant Massage Instructors. 1720 Willow Creek Cir. #516, Eugene, OR 97402. (800) 248-5432.

International Childbirth Education Association (ICEA). P.O. Box 20048, Minneapolis, MN 55420. (612) 854-8660, phone; (612) 854-8772, fax; info@icea.org, e-mail; http://www.icea.org, internet.

International Professional School of Bodywork. 1366 Hornblend Ave., San Diego, CA 92109. (858) 272-4142. Associates, bachelors, masters degrees in somatic practices. www.ipsbeing.com

Midwives' Alliance of North America (MANA). P.O. Box 175, Newton, KS 67114.

National Association of Childbirth Assistants (NACA). 936-B 7th St. #301, Novato, CA.

Prenatal and Postpartum Exercise Instructor Training by Elizabeth Noble, P.T. 48 Pleasant Lake Ave., Harwich, MA 02645. (508) 432-8040.

Rice Infant Sensorimotor Stimulation. Ruth D. Rice, Ph.D, Inc. 6455 Meadow Road, Dallas, Texas 75230.

Support and Referral

American Academy of Husband-Coached Childbirth (Bradley Method). P.O. Box 5224, Sherman Oaks, CA 91413.

American Diabetes Association. 1660 Duke St., Alexandria, VA 22314. (800) 232-3472.

American Heart Association. 7272 Greenville Ave., Dallas, TX 75231-4596. (800) 242-1793.

American Society for Psycho-Prophylaxis in Obstetrics, Inc (ASPO). 1200 19th St., NW #300, Washington, D.C. 20036-2422. (800) 368-4404. (Lamaze Method).

Back to Sleep. P.O. Box 29111, Washington, D.C. 20040. (800) 505-2742. Sudden Infant Death Syndrome (SIDS).

Center for Prevention of Sexual & Domestic Violence, 1914 N. 34th St., Suite 105, Seattle, WA 98103. (206) 634-1903.

Cesarean Prevention Movement, Inc. P.O. Box 152, Syracuse, NY 13210. (315) 424-1942.

Compassionate Friends. P.O. Box 3696, Oak Brook, IL 60522-3696. (708) 990-0010.

Home Oriented Maternity Experience (HOME). 511 New York Ave., Tacoma Park, Washington, D.C. 20012.

International Cesarean Awareness Network. 1647 W. 259th Pl., Harbor City, CA 90710.

La Leche League International. (Breastfeeding). 9616 Minneapolis Ave., Franklin Park, IL 60131.

National Association of Pregnancy Massage Therapy. Membership and therapist referrals: P.O. Box 9802-547, Austin, TX 78766-0802. (888) 451-4945.

National Council on Child Abuse and Family Violence. 1155 Connecticut Ave., NW, Suite 400, Washington, D.C. 20036. (202) 429-6695 or (800) 222-2000.

Postpartum Support International (PSI). 927 N. Kellogg Ave., Santa Barbara, CA 93111. (805) 967-7636.

Pre and Peri-natal Psychology Association of North America. 36 Madison Ave., Toronto, Ontario, M5R 251, Canada.

RTS Bereavement Services. 1910 South Avenue, La Crosse, WI 54601.

Vaginal Birth After Caesarean (VBAC). 10 Great Plain Terrace, Needham, Mass. 02192.

Bed rest:

Intensive Caring Unlimited (greater Philadelphia and southern New Jersey areas). 910 Bent Lane, Philadelphia, PA 19118. For referrals in Greater Philadelphia and surrounding counties, subscription information or resources: (215) 328-3128. For referrals in Southern New Jersey: (609) 799-2059.

The Confinement Line (Washington, D.C. area). C/O Childbirth Education Association, P.O. Box 1609, Springfield, VA 22151, (703) 941-7183.

High-Risk Moms, Inc. (greater Chicago area). P.O. Box 4013, Naperville, IL 60567-4013. (708) 357-5048.

Parent Care, Inc. (national organization). 101 1/2 South Union St., Alexandria, VA 22314. (703) 836-4678.

Sidelines National Support Network (high-risk and complicated pregnancies). P.O. Box 1808, Laguna Beach, CA 92652. (714) 497-2265.

Very Important Pregnancy Program (VIP) (bi-monthly newsletter). HealthDyne Perinatal Services, P.O. Box 11085, Rockford, IL 61126, (800) 999-2416, (800) 779-7676 (Ask-a-Nurse).

Recommended Reading for Practitioners and Mothers

Pregnancy & Childbirth:

Baldwin, Rahima and Terra Palarini. *Pregnant Feelings*. Celestial Arts: Berkeley, CA, 1986.

Burrow, Gerard N., M.D. and Thomas F. Ferris, M.D. *Medical Complications during Pregnancy, Third Edition*. W. B. Saunders: Philadelphia, PA, 1988.

Campbell, Leslie Kirk. *Journey Into Motherhood*. Riverhead Books: New York, 1996.

Dick-Read, Grantly, M.D. *Childbirth Without Fear*, Fifth Edition. Harper & Row: New York, 1984.

Gaskin, Ina May. *Spiritual Midwifery*. The Book Publishing Co.: Summerton, TN, 1978.

Gilbert, Elizabeth Stepp and Harmon, Judith Smith. *Manual of High Risk Pregnancy and Delivery*. Mosby: St. Louis, MO, 1993.

Harper, Barbara, RN. *Gentle Birth Choices*. Healing Arts Press: Rochester, VT, 1994.

Ilse, Sherokee. *Empty Arms: Coping with Miscarriage, Stillbirth & Infant Death*.

Jimenez, Sherry. *The Pregnant Woman's Comfort Guide*. Avery Publishing Group, Inc.: Garden City Park, New York, 1992.

Jones, Carl. *Mind Over Labor*. Penguin Books: New York, 1987.

Kitzinger, Sheila. *The Experience of Childbirth*. Third Edition. G. Nichols and Co.: London, 1974.

       The Complete Book of Pregnancy and Childbirth. Alfred A. Knopf: New York, 1990.

Leboyer, Frederick, M.D. *Birth Without Violence*. Knopf: New York, 1975.

McCutcheon, Susan. *Natural Childbirth the Bradley Way*. Revised Edition. Plumb: New York, 1996.

Moskowitz, Richard M.D. *Homeopathic Medicines for Pregnancy and Childbirth*. North Atlantic Books: Berkeley, CA, 1992.

Odent, Michel. *Birth Reborn*. Pantheon: New York, 1986.

Rich, Laurie A. *When Pregnancy Isn't Perfect*. Dutton: New York, 1991.

Rogers, Judith and Molleen, Matsumura. *Mother to Be: A Guide to Pregnancy and Birth For Women With Disabilities*. Demos Publications: New York, 1991.

Samuels, Mike, M.D., and Nancy. *The New Well Pregnancy Book*. Fireside Books: New York, 1996.

Simkin, Penny, P.T. *The Birth Partner*. Harvard Common Press: Boston, MA, 1989.

"Comfort Measures for Childbirth" video, Seattle, WA.

Simkin, Penny, Whalley, Janet, Keppler, Ann. *Pregnancy, Childbirth, and the Newborn: The Complete Guide*. Meadowbrook Press: Deephaven, 1991.

Massage & Movement:

CDR Communications, Inc. "Fundamentals of Therapeutic Massage: Body Mechanics" Video, #2 of 4 video series. Mosby Publishing: St. Louis, 1995.

Jones, Lawrence H., D.O. *Strain and Counterstrain*. The American Academy of Osteopathy: Newark, OH, 1981.

Klaus, Marshall H., M.D., Kennell, John H., M.D. , Klaus, Phyllis H., M.Ed. *Mothering the Mother: How a Doula Can Help You Have a Shorter, Easier, and Healthier Birth*. Addison-Wesley: New York, 1993.

Lieberman, Adrienne B. *Easing Labor Pain*. Harvard Common Press: Boston, MA, 1992.

Markowitz, Elysa and Howard Brainen. *Baby Dance: A Comprehensive Guide to Prenatal and Postpartum Exercise*. Prentice Hall, Inc.: Englewood Cliffs, New Jersey, 1980.

MedCom. "Massage for Pregnancy & Labor." Technical consultation by Carole Osborne-Sheets and others. Video.

Montagu, Ashley. *Touching: The Human Significance of the Skin*. Perennial Library, Harper & Row: New York, 1971.

Noble, Elizabeth, RPT. *Essential Exercises for the Childbearing Year*. 4th Edition. Houghton Mifflin Co.: Boston: MA, 1995.

Osborne-Sheets, Carole. *Deep Tissue Sculpting: A Technical and Artistic Manual for Therapeutic Bodywork Practitioners*. Poway, CA: Body Therapy Associates, 1990.

Osborne-Sheets, Carole. *Annotated Bibliography for Pre- and Perinatal Massage Therapy*. San Diego, CA, 1997.

Tappan, Francis M. *Healing Massage Techniques: Holistic, Classic, and Emerging Methods. Second Edition*. Appleton and Lange: Norwalk, CT, 1988.

Travell, Janet and Simons, D. *Myofascial Pain and Dysfunction, The Trigger Point Manual, the Lower Extremities, Volume 2*. Williams & Wilkins: Baltimore, MD, 1992.

Yates, John. *A Physician's Guide to Therapeutic Massage: Its Physiological Effects and their Application to Treatment*. Massage Therapists Association of B.C.: Vancouver, British Columbia, 1990. And others listed in Chapter Two endnotes, #8-28.

And others listed in Chapter Two endnotes, #8-28.

Parenting, Postpartum, Child Development and Massage:

Fleming Drehobl, Kathy and Gengler Ruhr, Mary. *Pediatric Massage For the Child with Special Needs*. Book and Video. Therapy Skill Builders: Tucson, AZ, 1991

Harrison, Helen. *The Premature Baby Book*. St. Martin's Press: New York, 1983.

Kitzinger, Sheila. *The Year After Childbirth*. Charles Scribner's Sons: New York, 1994.

Ourselves as Mothers. Addison-Wesley: New York, 1995.

Leboyer, Frederick, M.D. *Loving Hands*. Knopf: New York, 1979.

Levy, Janine. *The Baby Exercise Book for the First Fifteen Months*. Pantheon Books: New York, 1980.

Osborne-Sheets, Carole. *Massage Therapy and Movement for Infants*. Body Therapy Associates: San Diego, CA, 1998.

Rich, Adrienne. *Of Woman Born: Motherhood as Experience and Institution*. Norton: New York, 1976.

Schneider-McClure, Vimala. *Infant Massage: A Handbook for Loving Parents*. Bantam Books: Toronto, Ontario, 1982.

Sinclair, Marybetts. *Massage for Healthier Children*. Wingbow Press: Oakland, CA, 1992.

View Video. "Infant Massage: The Power of Touch" video, New York.

Index Words:

herpes, 37, 90, 120

hiatal hernia, 81

high-risk pregnancies, 50, 74

home births, 118

hormones, 4, 9, 33, 48, 56, 60, 96

hot packs, tubs, and baths, 42, 108, 111, 114, 117, 130

I

intrauterine growth retardation (small for gestational age), 11, 28-29, 31, 37, 39, 41, 44, 47, 52-53, 65-66, 83

indigestion, 10

infant massage, 23-24, 92, 94, 134, 138 (also see maternal touch)

intrauterine pressure, 11, 28-29, 31, 37, 41, 53, 65-66, 83

K

Kegel, 12, 19, 62, 77, 89-90, 93-94, 138 (also see pelvic floor)

L

labor and birth

"back labor", 113-114, 117, 122, 124

contractions, 21, 34, 36-38, 40, 46, 49, 56, 59, 80-81, 88, 90, 98-110, 112-117, 119, 121-124, 127, 130, 142-143

dilation, 16, 81, 99-101, 104, 107, 111, 115-116

effacement, 81, 99-101, 115-116

heat and cold, 108, 111, 114, 117

fetal positions, 14-15, 111

"laboring mind", 109-110

massage techniques, 11, 23, 35, 37, 42, 55, 76, 78, 90-93, 117, 122, 140

pain, 18, 20, 59, 76, 83, 97, 106, 108, 118-120, 126-127, 145

physiology, 27, 138, 148

positions, 19, 28, 89, 91, 94, 102, 106, 109-110, 112, 117-118, 124, 126-127, 146

practitioners' care, 34

precautions, 134, 144

preparation, 5, 13, 18-19, 77, 82-83, 88-91, 93-95, 105

prolonged, 3, 117, 120

scope of practice, 12, 42, 61, 76, 111, 138

sounding, 124

stages, 100, 105, 137 (also see cesarean birth, emotions)

ligamentous laxity, 13-14, 30, 41, 73, 77, 80

lupus, 36, 39, 52-53

M

maternal touch, 22-23, 26

medications

anesthesia, 20-21,25-26, 29, 96, 106, 118, 126, 129, 136, 144

epidural, 21, 107, 141

pitocin, 106-107, 126, 130

membranes (amniotic) 37, 44, 46-47, 52, 98

multiple gestations, 36, 51

musculoskelatal structures

adductor, 7, 18, 91-93, 101, 116-118, 124

erector spinae, 62, 78, 93, 101, 108, 142

gastrocnemius/soleus, 16, 72-73, 94

gluteus medius, maximus, 13, 71, 142

hamstrings, 91, 93

hip joint, 7, 12, 16, 18, 42, 93, 143

iliocostalis, 71

iliopsoas, 12, 25, 72, 77, 80, 84, 93, 134, 142-143

infraspinatus, 13

inguinal ligament, 7

intercostals, 10, 87

intrinsic spinal extensors and rotators, 72, 78

levator scapula, 10, 62, 78, 93, 101, 148

longisimus, 71

lumbosacral joint, 12, 14, 28, 78, 83-84, 93, 108, 111

masseter, 101, 113

pectoralis major, 10, 62, 78, 86, 93

pectoralis minor, 10, 62, 78, 93

perineum, 90, 104, 118, 128 (also see pelvic floor)

peroneals, 16

piriformis, 16, 18, 71, 95, 138, 142

psoas, 80, 96

pubic symphysis, 14, 141

quadratus lumborum, 71, 101, 138, 142, 147-148

rectus abdominus, 12, 80, 88, 133

rectus femoris, 7

rhomboidei, 62, 78, 148

sacroiliac joint, 12-14, 28, 30, 66, 70, 78-79, 83, 85, 93, 111, 126, 134

sartorius, 7, 39, 43

11650 Iberia Place #137 ♦ San Diego, CA 92128
Phone: 800-586-8322 ♦ Fax: 858-748-8827 ♦ www.bodytherapyassociates.com
Visit our secure website for on-line orders and class registrations.

Product List

Quantity	Titles by Carole Osborne-Sheets	Price	Total
	Annotated Bibliography	15.00	
	Deep Tissue Sculpting: Second Edition	21.95	
	Pre- & Perintal Massage Therapy	24.95	
	Interviews & Articles Collection	5.00	
	Massage Therapy & Movement for Infants: A Therapist's Handbook	10.00	
	Other Books and Supplies		
	Birth Partner by P. Simkin	12.95	
	Breast Massage by Debra Curtus	36.95	
	Essential Exercises for the Childbearing Year by E. Noble	16.95	
	Infant Massage: A Handbook for Loving Parents by V. Schneider-McClure	14.95	
	Massage for Healthier Children by M. Sinclair	15.95	
	Physician's Guide to Therapeutic Massage by J. Yates	12.95	
	The New Well Pregnancy Book by M. and N. Samuels	20.00	
	When Pregnancy Isn't Perfect by Laurie Rich	18.95	
	Maternal Love CD	10.95	
	Prenatal Support Pillow	14.50	
	Infant Massage: The Power of Touch video tape	19.95	
	Tai Chi for Health video tape	19.98	
	Comfort Measures for Childbirth with Penny Simkin videotape	39.95	
	Contoured bodyCushion® by Body Support Systems	varies	

Shipping:

	Priority	Book Rate
$0 - $25	$ 7.90	$3.60
$26 - $47	$ 9.85	$5.60
$48+	$11.05	$7.60

Please allow 3-4 days for Priority Shipping;
1-2 weeks for Book Rate

Product Subtotal _____

Shipping & Handling (see chart) _____

Tax (CA residents only, add 7.75 %) _____

Total _____

PRICE AND AVAILABILITY SUBJECT TO CHANGE
CREDIT CARD, CHECK OR MONEY ORDER — MAKE PAYABLE TO BODY THERAPY ASSOCIATES

Name: _____

Address: _____

Phone: _____ ☐ Visa ☐ Master Card ☐ Amex # _____ Exp. _____

Please send information and schedule of workshops for:

☐ Certification in Pre- & Perinatal Massage Therapy

☐ Introduction to Rhythmic Deep Tissue Sculpting